Instant Pot Recipes

The Tastiest Instant Pot Recipes Around

Jessica Moore

Table of Contents

thought of as universal. As befitting its nature, it is presented without assurance regarding its prolonged validity or interim quality. Trademarks that are mentioned are done without written consent and can in no way be considered an endorsement from the trademark holder.

Introduction

Congratulations on purchasing *Instant Pot Recipes*. Thank you so much for doing so!

Take a moment to think about your current eating habits; more than likely you quickly snag an energy bar on the way out the door in the morning. There are many times during the course of an average workday that you make friends with the vending machine. And after a long day at work and then rounding up the kids from school and assisting with homework, the last thing you want to be doing is cooking a meal that includes the time to prep, cook, and wash dishes afterward. You are more than likely used to having your favorite fast food joint doing the hard work for you when it comes to dinnertime. But do we really know the havoc we are wreaking on our health?

Even though there is never enough hours in the day, in today's world it is now more possible than ever to make and create delicious, homemade meals in the comfort of our own kitchen that are not only easy to whip up but healthy as well. If you have stumbled across this book, you more than likely already know the star of this cookbook pretty well (well, I would hope). The instant pot is a contraption that is wildly underestimated when it comes to discovering meals that are not only simple to make but also fuel your body in positive ways.

Yes, there are indeed a plethora of instant pot cookbooks and other resources out there that provide homemakers a variety of recipes. But I guarantee this is one of the healthiest instant pot cookbooks you will come across! It was written with the health conscious in mind. We all know what it is like to finally want to take steps that lead to creating the best versions of ourselves. Now you can with the wide array of delectable, healthy recipes in this cookbook!

Thanks again for purchasing this cookbook! Every effort was made to ensure it is full of as much useful and tasty recipes as possible, please enjoy!

Breakfast Recipes

3-Minute Oats

What's in it:

- 3 C. water
- 1 C. steel cut oats

How it's made:

- Put oats into your instant pot. Pour in 3 cups of water.
- Cover. Push MANUAL and set timer 3 minutes.
- Let instant pot pressurize for 5 minutes.
- Perform natural release for 5-10 minutes.
- Garnish with toppings of choice and enjoy!

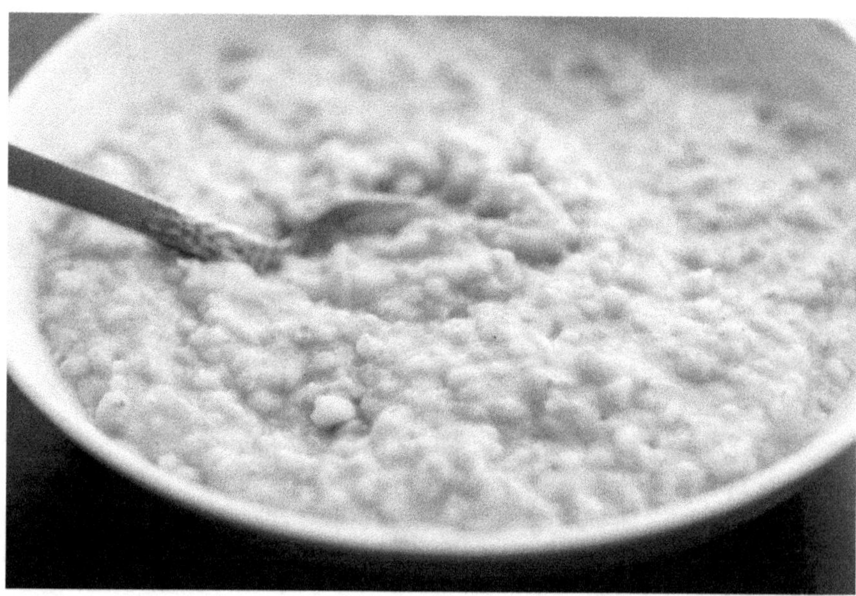

Banana French Toast

What's in it:

- ¼ C. chopped pecans
- 2 tbsp. sliced/chilled butter
- ½ tsp. cinnamon
- 1 tsp. vanilla extract
- 1 tbsp. sugar
- ½ C. almond milk
- 3 eggs
- ¼ C. cream cheese
- 2 tbsp. light brown sugar
- 4 sliced bananas
- 5-6 cubed slices of French bread

How it's made:

- Grease a dish that fits in your instant pot.
- Cut French bread into cubes. Place a layer of bread into the dish. Then layer banana slices with a few sprinkles of brown sugar.
- Melt cream cheese in microwave for 30 seconds until creamy. Pour over bananas.
- Place remaining bread into dish and layer with remaining bananas and brown sugar. Pour half of the pecans over the top.
- Beat eggs with cinnamon, vanilla, sugar, and almond milk. Pour egg mixture into dish over bread.
- Pour about ¾ cup of water into the bottom of the instant pot. Put a trivet over water and gently place the dish on a trivet.
- Cover. Set timer for 25 minutes on HIGH PRESSURE.
- Release pressure by venting.

- Allow mixture to sit 5 minutes and then top with maple syrup, remaining nuts, and bananas.

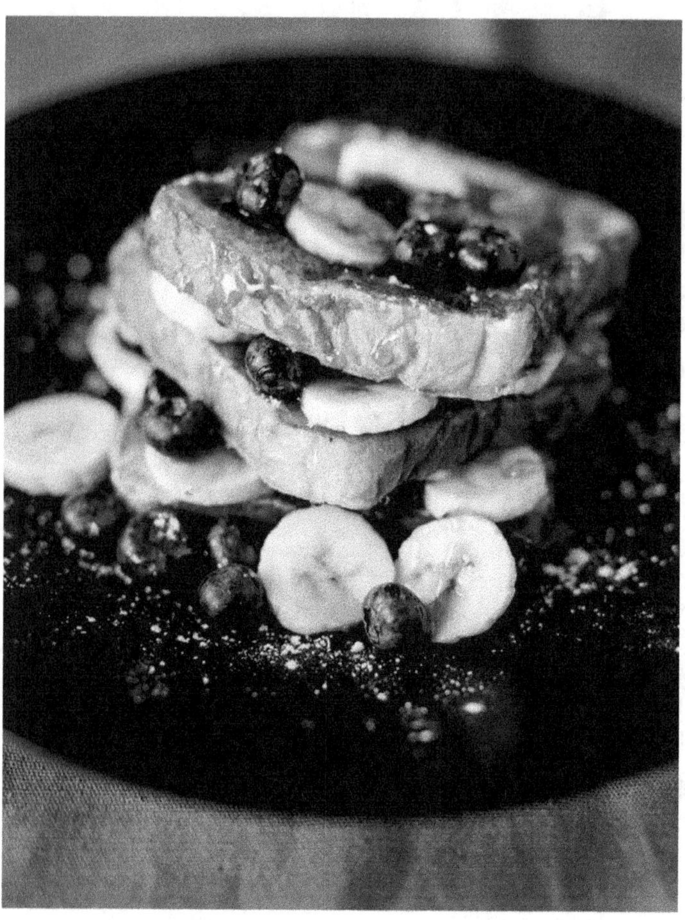

Ham, Egg, and Cheese Casserole

What's in it:

- 1 tsp. pepper
- 1 tsp. salt
- 1 C. almond milk
- 10-12 eggs
- 2 C. shredded cheddar cheese
- 1 diced onion
- 1-2 C. chopped ham
- 32 ounces frozen hash browns

How it's made:

- Grease instant pot insert.
- Place half of hash browns into bottom of the pot. Top with 1/3 of cheese, ham, and onions. Repeat this step twice, layering these ingredients.
- Beat pepper, salt, milk, and eggs together. Then pour over layers in the pot.
- Push SLOW COOKER and then the ADJUST button. Set to 7 hours.

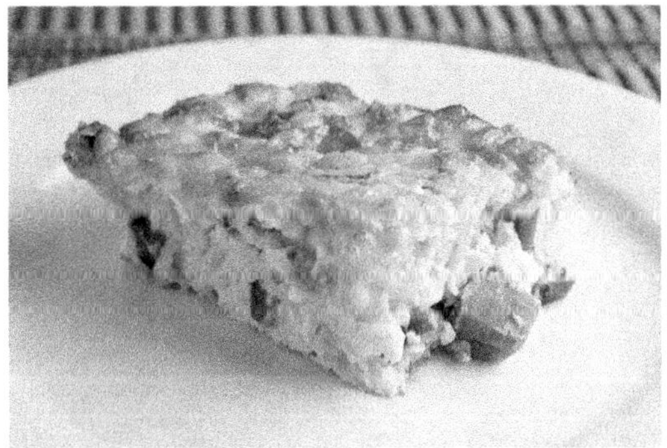

Egg Muffins

What's in it:

- 4 slices cooked/crumbled bacon
- 1 diced green onion
- 4 tbsp. shredded cheddar cheese
- ¼ tsp. lemon pepper seasoning
- 4 eggs

How it's made:

- Place a steamer basket into your instant pot and pour in 1 ½ cups of water.
- Beat eggs and lemon pepper together.
- Split up green onion, bacon, and cheese between 4 muffin cups. Pour lemon-egg mixture into cups and stir.
- Put cups into the steamer basket.
  Cover and push HIGH. Set to cook 8 minutes.
- When the timer goes off, turn off the pot and wait 2-3 minutes and perform a quick pressure release.
- Take out muffin cups and enjoy!

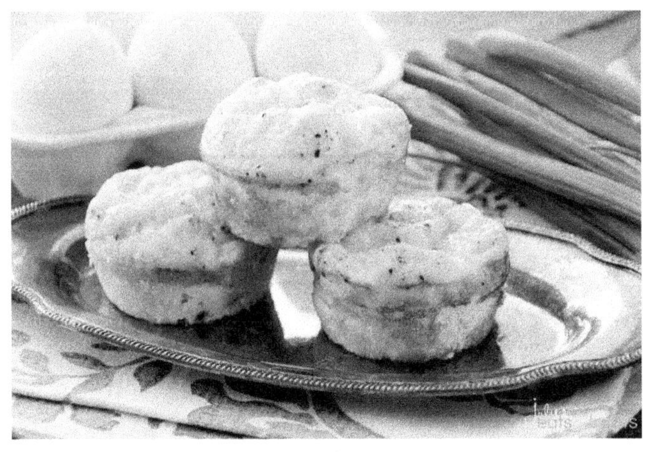

Instant Pot Strawberry Jam

What's in it:

- 1 C. raw honey
- 1 pound diced strawberries

How it's made:

- Turn on the instant pot to SAUTE and pour in honey. Let it melt till you can stir it with ease. Add strawberries.
- Bring mixture to a boil. When bubbles begin to turn pink, cover and set to HIGH PRESSURE, cooking 3 minutes. Perform natural release.
- Uncover and mash strawberries.
- Turn instant pot to SAUTE to boil the excess liquid. Once the mixture is able to coat the back of a spoon, jam is ready.
- Let cool to room temp. Store in fridge.

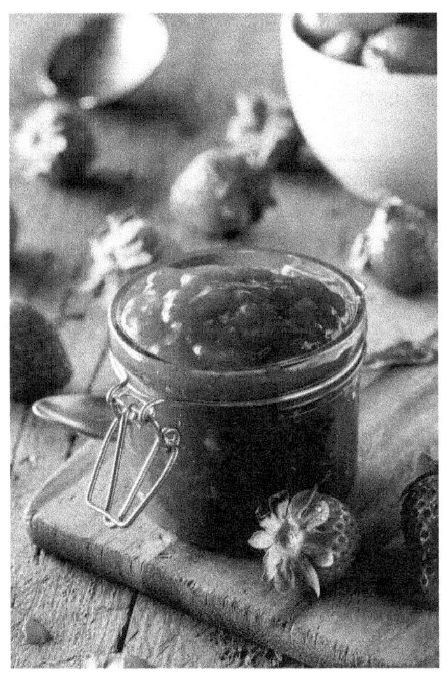

5-Ingredient Cheesy Egg Bake

What's in it:

- ½ tsp. pepper
- 1 tsp. salt
- ½ C. shredded cheddar cheese
- ¼ C. milk
- 6 eggs
- 2 C. frozen hash browns
- 6 slices chopped bacon

How it's made:

- Chop bacon into pieces and sauté in instant pot until crisp. If you would like veggies, add to bacon and sauté 3 minutes.
- Pour in hash browns and cook 2 minutes till thawed.
- Grease metal container that fits in instant pot.
- Whisk pepper, salt, cheese, milk, and eggs together. Add bacon mixture and combine. Pour egg mixture into the greased container.
- Place 1 ½ cups of water into the bottom of the instant pot. Place a trivet over water and gently place the container on a trivet.
- Cover. Set on HIGH PRESSURE and set to cook 10 minutes. Perform quick release.
- Loosen edges and place onto a serving plate.
- Serve with additional cheese.

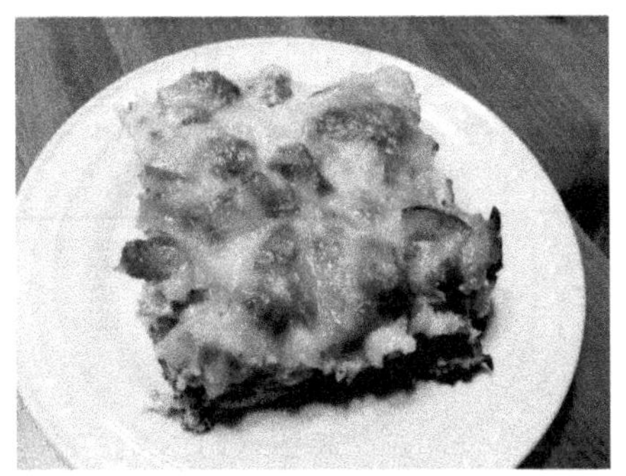

Crust-Less Meat Lover's Quiche

What's in it:

- 1 C. shredded cheese of choice
- 2 chopped green onions
- ½ C. diced ham
- 1 C. cooked ground sausage
- 4 cooked/crumbled bacon
- 1/8 tsp. pepper
- ¼ tsp. salt
- ½ C. almond milk
- 6 beaten eggs

How it's made:

- Place trivet into the bottom of the instant pot. Pour in 1 cup of water.
- Whisk pepper, salt, milk, and eggs together. Then stir in cheese, green onions, ham, sausage, and bacon till combined. Pour mixture into a dish.
- Place dish upon trivet within the instant pot.
- Set to cook 30 minutes on HIGH PRESSURE.
- When timer beeps, wait 10 minutes then perform a quick release.
- Sprinkle quiche with additional cheese and broil until melted if desired.

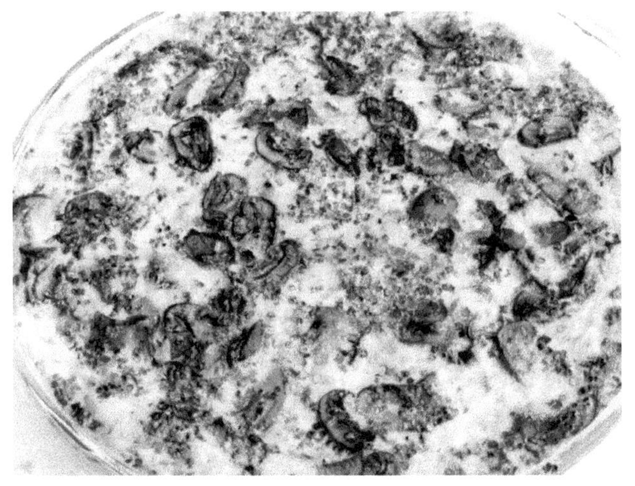

Twice Baked Potato Casserole

What's in it:

- 4 sliced cooked/crumbled bacon
- 1 chopped bundle green onions
- 2 C. shredded cheddar cheese + more for topping
- 1 ranch seasoning packet
- 1 C. low-fat sour cream
- 1 C. almond milk
- Pepper and salt
- 1 ½ sticks butter
- 5 pounds potatoes of choice

How it's made:

- Slice potatoes into chunks, leaving skin attached. Place into the instant pot with 1 stick of butter, a cup of water, pepper, and salt.
- Cover and set to MANUAL to cook 6 minutes.
- Perform quick release. Then add in almond milk and remaining butter.
- Combine with electric mixer or potato masher. Then stir in ranch seasoning and sour cream till well incorporated.
- Mix in green onions and cheddar cheese.
- Transfer mixture to a dish. Top with bacon, chives, and additional cheese.
- Bake 20 minutes at 350 degrees. Enjoy!

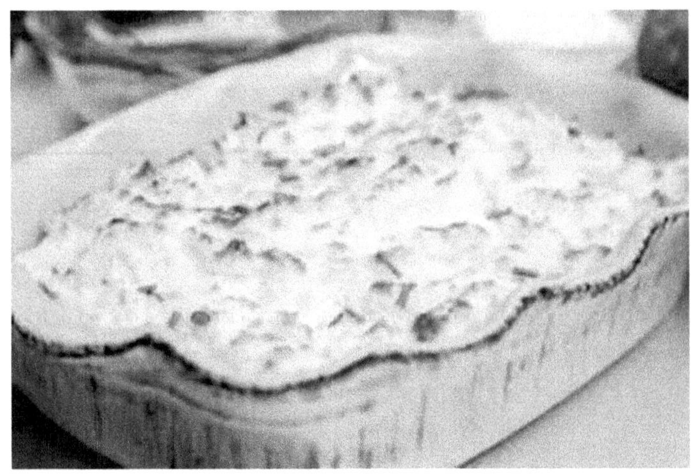

Mexican Egg Casserole

What's in it:

- 1 C. mozzarella cheese
- 1 C. Cotija cheese
- ½ C. flour
- ½ C. green onions
- 1 can black beans
- 1 chopped red bell pepper
- ½ chopped red onion
- 1 pound ground sausage
- 8 beaten eggs
- Cilantro
- Sour cream

How it's made:

- Sauté onion and sausage together in instant pot for 5-6 minutes till meat is thoroughly cooked.
- Mix eggs and flour together and pour into egg mixture. Then place cheeses, beans, and chopped veggies into the instant pot. Reserve a bit of mozzarella cheese for serving.
- Cover and set to HIGH to cook 20 minutes. Perform natural release.
- Sprinkle with remaining cheese and let sit for a few minutes till melted. Serve with sour cream and devour!

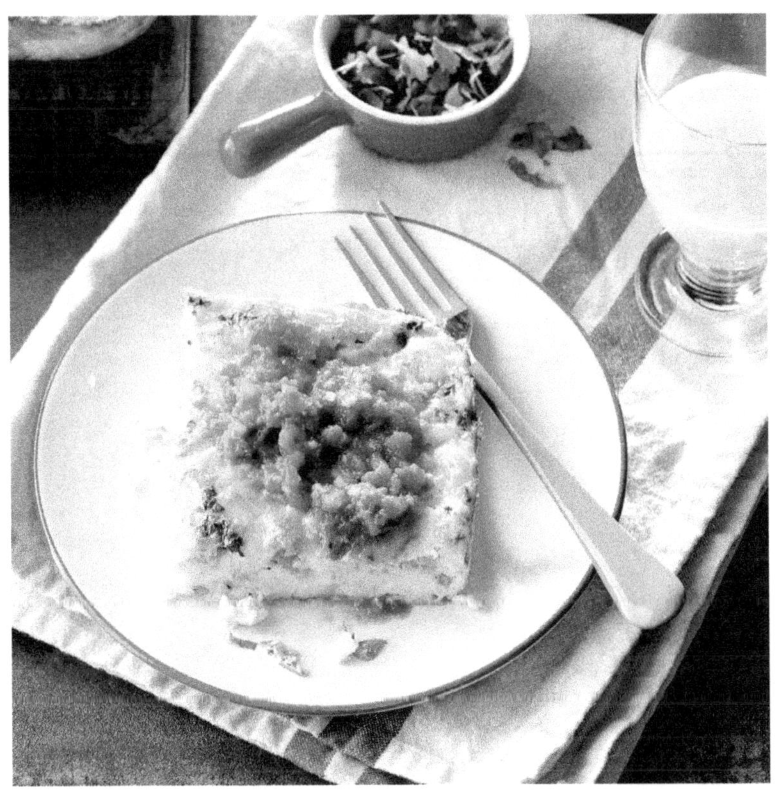

Cuban Potato Egg Frittata

What's in it:

- 1 ½ C. water
- 4 ounces shredded cheese of choice
- 1 tsp. tomato paste
- ¼ C. almond milk
- 2 tbsp. bisquick
- 1 minced clove garlic
- 1 tsp. seasoning of choice
- ¼ tsp. pepper
- ½ tsp. salt
- ¼ C. diced scallions
- 1 tbsp. melted butter
- 4 ounces hash browns
- 6 eggs
- 1 ounce grated cheese of choice, for topping

Optional Add-ins:

- Sausage
- Ham
- Spinach
- Bacon
- Bell pepper

How it's made:

- Soak hash browns in water 30 minutes.
- Whisk seasonings and eggs together till combined.
- Mix milk, tomato paste, and Bisquick together and then combine with egg mixture.

- Take hash browns out of water and pat with paper towels. Combine with melted butter. Combine with egg mixture.
- Pour egg and hash brown mixture into a dish and top with cheese.
- Place a trivet into your instant pot and pour in water. Gently put dish upon trivet.
- Cover and set to cook 15-20 minutes on HIGH PRESSURE.
- Perform a 10-minute natural release.
- Top with cheese and allow time for the cheese to become gooey.

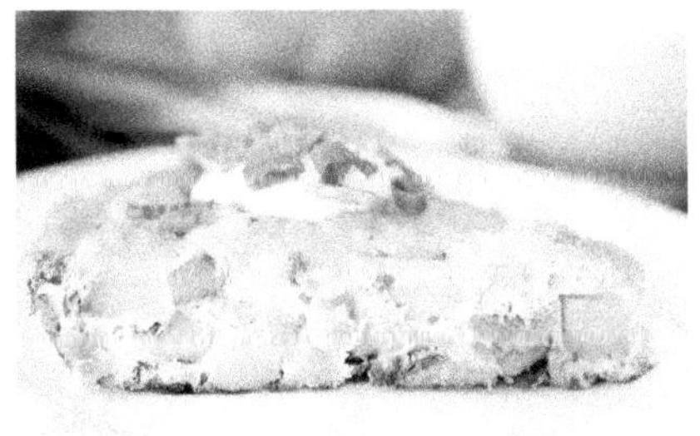

pple and Squash Breakfast Porridge

What's in it:

- 1/8 tsp. cloves
- 1/8 tsp. ginger
- Pinch of salt
- 2 tbsp. maple syrup
- 2 tbsp. gelatin
- ½ C. bone broth
- 1 delicata squash
- 4 small apples of choice

How it's made:

- Put whole squash into your instant pot. Slice apples into chunks and add to pot. Then pour in spices and bone broth, stirring well to combine.
- Cover and set to cook 8 minutes on MANUAL. Perform natural release for 10 minutes the push CANCEL.
- Put squash on a plate and slice in half lengthwise. Take out seeds and put into a blender.
- Pour remaining mixture of the instant pot into a blender with squash and add remaining recipe components. Blend 30 seconds till smooth.
- Serve with toppings of choice.

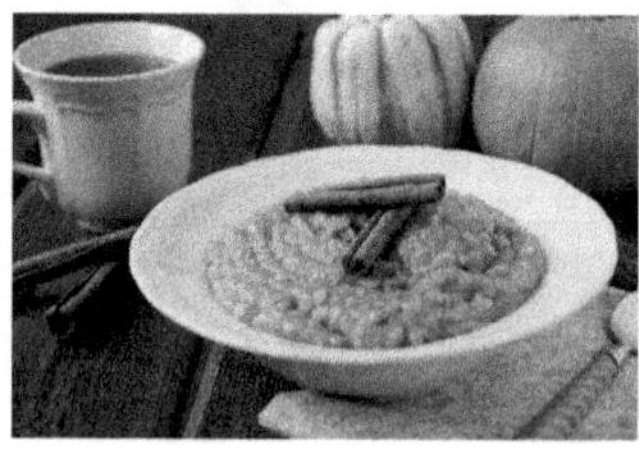

Lunch Recipes

Red Beans and Rice

What's in it:

- 10 C. cooked rice
- 1 pound chicken sausage (cut thinly into slices)
- 7 C. water
- 2 bay leaves
- ½ tsp. thyme
- 1 tsp. hot sauce
- ¼ tsp. white pepper
- ½ tsp. black pepper
- 1 tsp. salt
- 1 pound dry red kidney beans
- 3 diced stalks celery
- 1 diced bell pepper
- 1 diced onion

How it's made:

- Place all recipe components minus rice and sausage into the instant pot.
- Cover and set to cook 28 minutes on HIGH PRESSURE.
- Perform quick release.
- Add sausage and recover pot. Set to cook 15 minutes on MANUAL. Perform a quick release.
- Allow mixture to sit 10-15 minutes to thicken. Serve over cooked rice and enjoy!

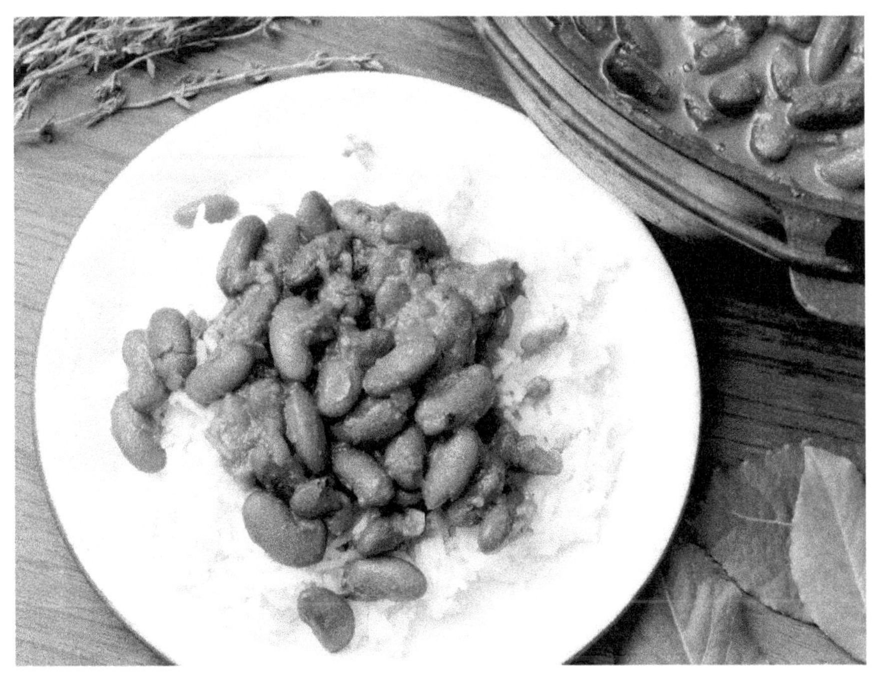

Tavern Sandwiches

What's in it:

- 8 slices American cheese
- 1 tbsp. ketchup
- 2 tbsp. mustard
- 10 ¾ ounces tomato soup
- 10 ¾ ounces chicken gumbo soup
- ¼ tsp. pepper
- ½ tsp. salt
- 3 chopped green onions
- 2 pounds ground beef
- Sandwich buns

How it's made:

- Cook ground beef within instant pot set to SAUTE mode. Cook till no longer pink and drain grease.
- Add in remaining recipe components, minus the cheese. Set to cook 7 minutes on MANUAL.
- Perform quick release.
- Serve beef mixture on top of buns and topped with a slice of cheese. Enjoy!

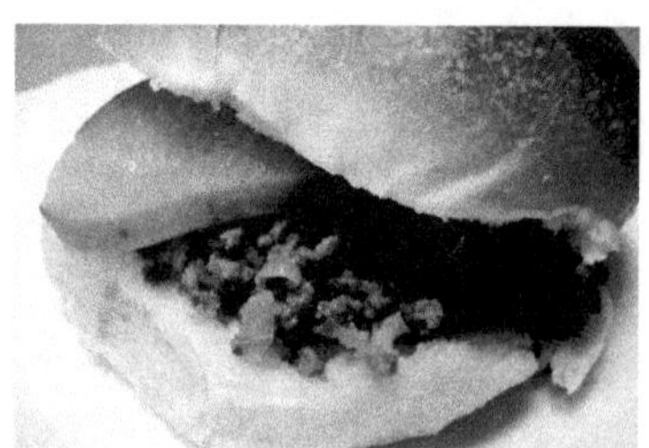

Instant Pot Beef Gyros

What's in it:

- 4 tbsp. olive oil
- 1 tbsp. lemon juice
- 1 sliced red onion
- ½ C. vegetable broth
- 1 tsp. salt
- 1 tsp. pepper
- 1 tbsp. dried parsley
- 3 minced cloves garlic
- 2 pounds thinly sliced beef roasted
- Pita bread

Tzatziki Sauce:

- 2 tbsp. dill
- 1 tsp. pepper and salt
- 1 minced clove garlic
- ½ C. cucumber
- 1 C. Greek yogurt

Optional Toppings:

- Lettuce
- Cucumbers
- Onions
- Carrots
- Feta or goat cheese

How it's made:

- Sauté garlic, onion, meat, and seasonings in your instant pot till onions are soft.
- Add in broth and lemon juice.
  Cover and set to cook 9 minutes on MEAT/STEW setting.
- Perform natural release for 3 minutes.
- Mix up sauce ingredients and slice optional toppings.
- Serve meat over pita bread, topped with tzatziki sauce and optional toppings.

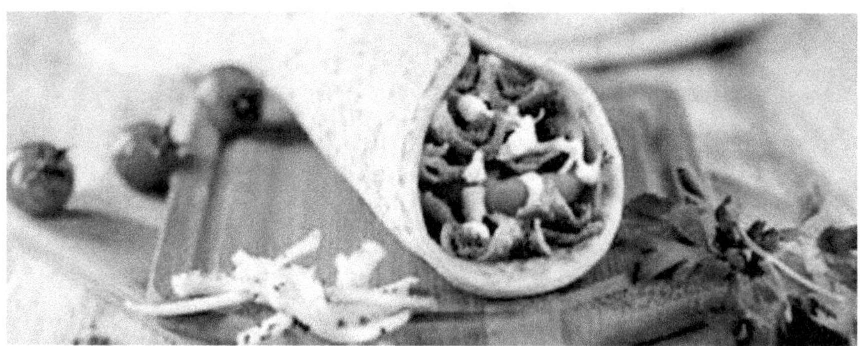

Kielbasa with Sauerkraut and Potatoes

What's in it:

- 3 tbsp. olive oil
- ½ tsp. pepper
- ½ tsp. salt
- 1 C. diced onion
- 1-2 diced potatoes
- 2-3 C. sauerkraut
- 1 pound beef, chicken, or turkey kielbasa (sliced in 1" chunks)
- 2 C. water

How it's made:

- Warm up oil on SAUTE mode in instant pot. Sauté onions and potatoes together until softened. Press CANCEL to turn the pot off.
- Pour in water and sauerkraut, stir well to combine.
- Layer kielbasa slices over potatoes.
- Cook 5 minutes on STEAM.
- Perform quick release.
- Serve!

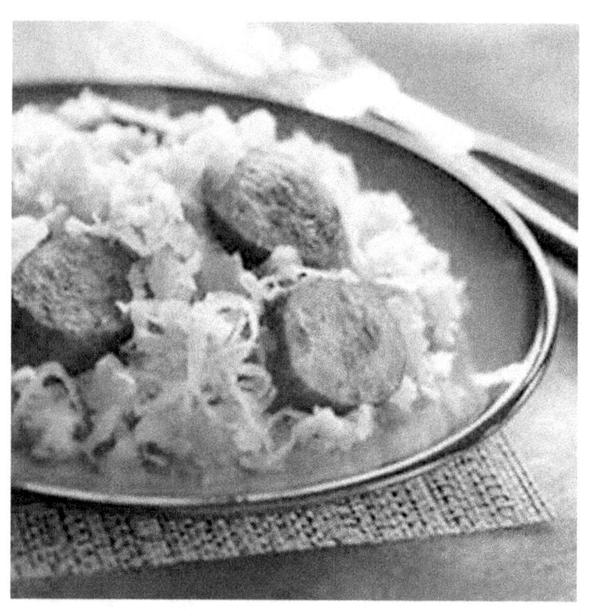

Hawaiian Fried Rice

What's in it:

- 1 C. chopped pineapple
- 2 tbsp. soy sauce
- 2 C. water
- 1 ½ C. brown rice
- 3 lightly scrambled eggs
- 2 C. cooked/cubed ham
- 1 chopped red bell pepper
- 1 diced onion
- 1 tbsp. olive oil

- Chopped scallions (serving)

How it's made:

- Sauté red pepper, onion, and olive onion together in instant pot until soft. Then stir in ham. Pour in beaten eggs, stirring till cooked through.
- Add pineapple, soy sauce, water, and brown rice. Cover and cook 24 minutes on MANUAL.
- Keep on WARM 5 minutes.
- Serve garnished with scallions. Enjoy!

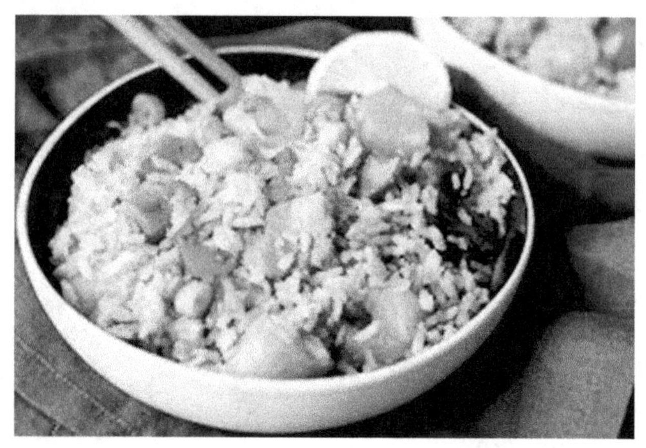

Instant Pot Mac n' Cheese

What's in it:

- 8 ounces shredded Monterey jack cheese
- 8 ounces shredded sharp cheddar cheese
- 12-ounce can evaporated milk
- 3-4 dashes hot sauce
- 1 tbsp. salt
- 1 tbsp. Dijon mustard
- 2 tbsp. butter
- 4 C. water
- 1 pound pasta shells or macaroni noodles

How it's made:

- Combine hot sauce, salt, mustard, butter, water, and pasta together in your instant pot insert. Cover and cook 4 minutes on HIGH PRESSURE.
- Perform quick release. Turn off the instant pot.
- Stir in shredded cheeses and evaporated milk. Keep stirring until cheeses melt.

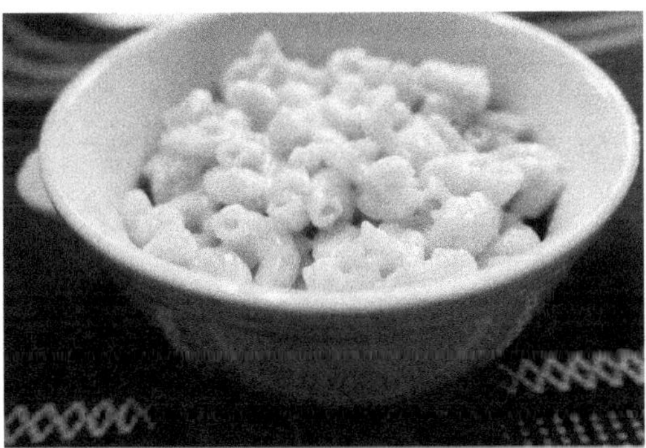

Potato Salad

What's in it:

- Pepper and salt
- 1 tbsp. mustard
- 1 tbsp. dill pickle juice
- 2 tbsp. chopped parsley
- 1 C. mayo
- 4 eggs
- ¼ C. chopped onion
- 1 ½ C. water
- 6 peeled/cubed russet potatoes

How it's made:

- Place a steamer basket into your instant pot.
- Pour in water and then add eggs and potatoes.
- Set to cook 4 minutes on HIGH PRESSURE.
- Perform quick release.
- Place eggs in ice cold water.
- Mix together mustard, pickle juice, parsley, mayo, and onion. Mix in cooled potatoes and gently combine.
- Peel and cut up eggs and add to salad. Season with pepper and salt.
- Chill for an hour before preparing to serve. Enjoy!

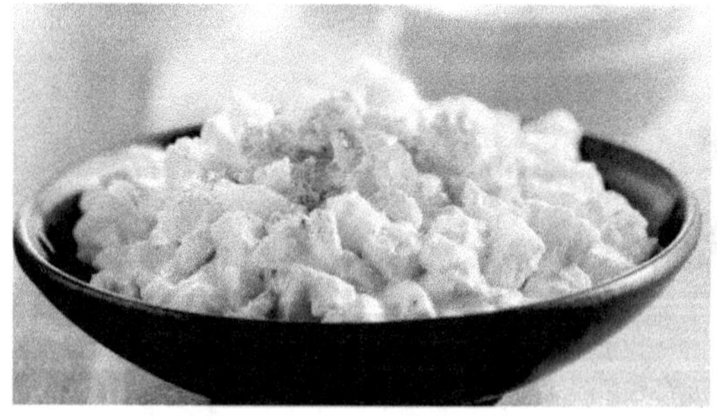

Chicken Burrito Bowls

What's in it:

- 1 C. salsa
- Chili powder
- Pepper and salt
- 2 pounds boneless chicken breasts

- Toppings of choice: Cheese, scallions, sour cream, etc.)

How it's made:

- Place chicken into the bottom of the instant pot. Season with pepper, salt, and chili powder. Pour salsa over chicken.
- Cover and set to cook 7 minutes on MANUAL.
- Perform quick release.
- Take out chicken and shred. Top meat with cooking liquids and stir well.
- Place into bowls and top with garnishes of choice.

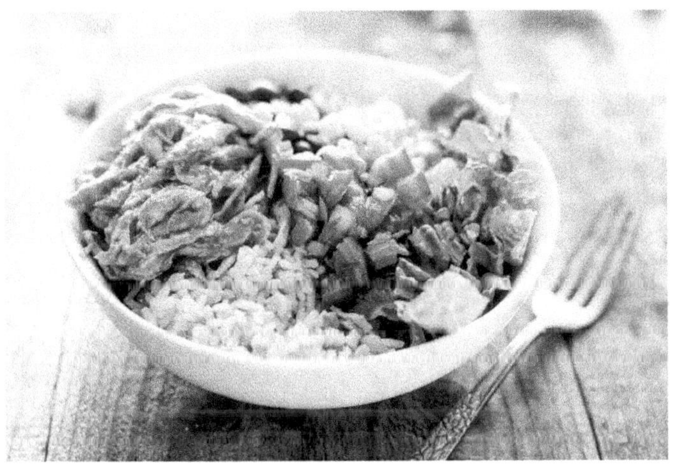

Pizza Pull-Apart Bread

What's in it:

- 1 package mini pepperonis
- 4 minced cloves garlic
- 2 tbsp. chopped parsley
- 2 C. mozzarella cheese
- 1/3 C. olive oil
- 2 cans pizza dough
- Pizza sauce, for serving

How it's made:

- Slice pizza dough into 1-inch by 2-inch strips.
- Combine remaining recipe components together, minus pizza sauce. Mix together with dough strips with hands till incorporated.
- Place strips into a pan that fits in instant pot.
- Pour a cup of water into the bottom of the pot. Place pan gently within the pot.
- Cook 10 minutes on HIGH PRESSURE. Perform a quick release.
- Serve with warmed up pizza sauce as a dip!

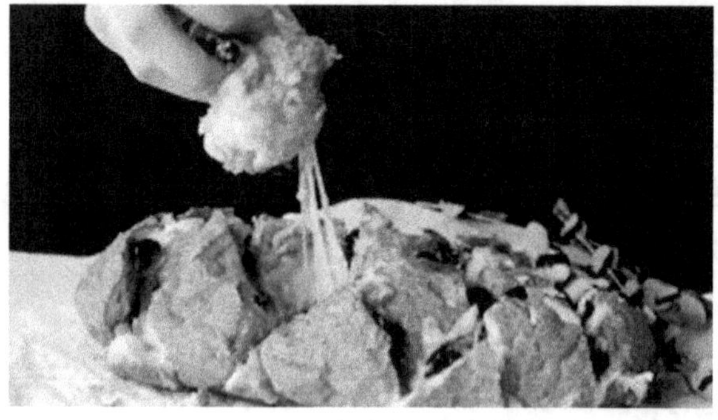

20-Minute Jacket Potato

What's in it:

- Pepper and salt
- 1 tbsp. butter
- 4 potatoes of choice

How it's made:

- Pour 1 cup of water into the bottom of your instant pot.
- With a fork, prick potatoes and season liberally with pepper and salt.
- Put steamer rack in instant pot and place potatoes into the rack.
- Cover and cook 20 minutes on STEAM.
- Serve warm with toppings of choice!

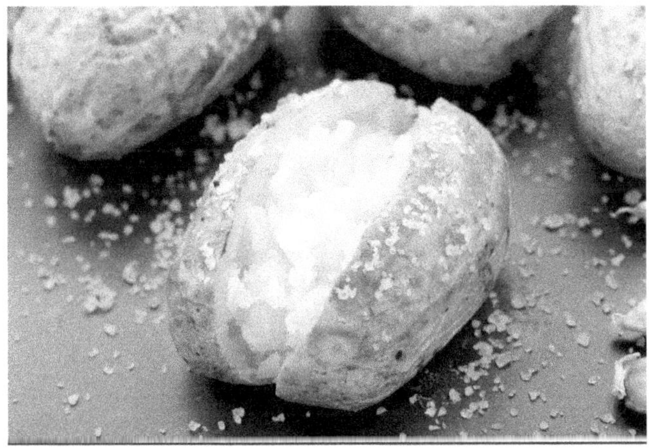

Soup Recipes

Lemon Chicken Noodle Soup

What's in it:

- ½ C. chopped parsley
- 1 tsp. herbs d' province
- 1 tsp. thyme
- 1-2 zested and juiced lemon
- 2 ½ C. whole wheat egg noodles
- 6 C. low-sodium chicken broth
- 2 trimmed chicken breasts
- 2 minced cloves garlic
- ¾ tsp. salt
- Pepper
- 1 bundle chopped green onions
- 1 C. chopped celery
- 3 C. chopped carrots

How it's made:

- Grease metal insert with olive oil.
- Sauté carrots, celery, and green onions (whites and green portions) together. Season with 1/8 tsp pepper and salt. Sauté till carrots are browned.
- Add garlic and cook 60 seconds. Then pour in broth, ½ tsp. salt, pepper, and place chicken breasts into the mixture.
- Cover and set to MANUAL to cook 15 minutes.
- Perform quick release. Remove chicken.
- Add in pasta. Recover and set MANUAL to cook for 0 minutes.
- Shred chicken with forks as pasta cooks.
- Once pasta is done, perform quick release and add shredded chicken back into the instant pot.

- Stir in parsley, herbs d' province, lemon juice, lemon zest, and thyme.

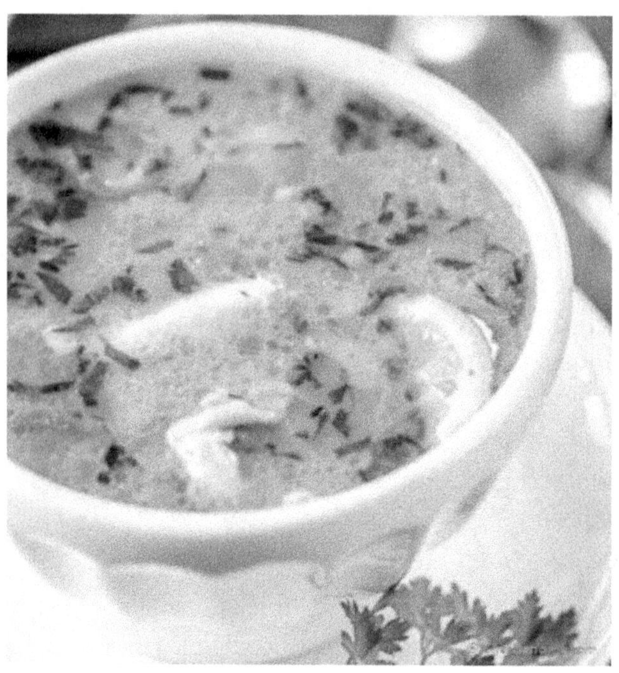

Butternut Cauliflower Soup

What's in it:

- ½ C. half and half
- ¼ tsp. salt
- ¼ - ½ tsp. red pepper flakes
- ½ - 1 tsp. dried thyme
- 1 tsp. paprika
- 2 C. vegetable broth
- 1 pound cubed butternut squash
- 1 pound cauliflower
- 2-3 minced cloves garlic
- 1-2 tsp. olive oil
- 1 diced onion

Topping Options:

- Pesto
- Croutons
- Sunflower seeds
- Pumpkin seeds
- Chopped green onions
- Sour cream
- Cheddar, parmesan, and/or mozzarella cheese
- Chives
- Sriracha or hot sauce
- Crumbled bacon

How it's made:

- Sauté onion with olive oil within instant pot until tender. Add garlic at the end of sautéing onion.

- Then add spices, vegetable broth, butternut squash, and cauliflower. Stir well.
- Set to cook 5 minutes on HIGH PRESSURE. Perform a quick release.
- Mix in half and half and blend mixture with an immersion blender until creamy and smooth.
- Top soup with choice of toppings and enjoy!

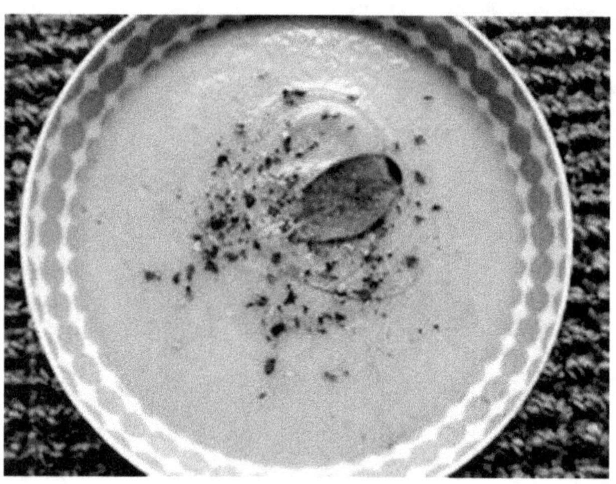

Low-Carb Beef Soup

What's in it:

- 2 cans beef broth
- 2 can diced tomatoes
- ½ pound green beans
- 1 tsp. oregano
- 1 tsp. thyme
- 1 tbsp. minced garlic
- 1 chopped onion
- 1 pound lean beef
- 1 tsp. olive oil
- Pepper and salt
- Grated parmesan cheese

How it's made:

- Warm up oil in instant pot and sauté onion with beef till cooked. Then add in oregano, thyme, and garlic and cook 3 minutes.
- Pour in broth and tomatoes with juice.
- Trim green beans and cut into 1" pieces. Add to instant pot.
- Clover and cook 30 minutes on LOW PRESSURE. Perform quick release.
- Season with pepper and salt and serve topped with grated parmesan cheese.

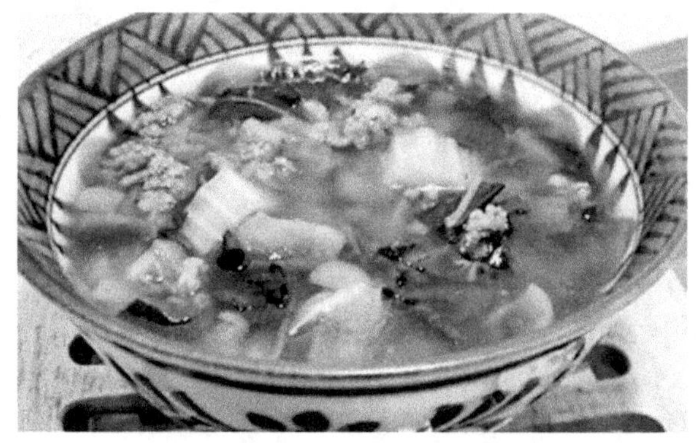

Taco Soup

What's in it:

- 15 ounces canned pinto beans
- 3 1/3 ounces diced tomatoes with green chilies
- 5 1/8 ounces canned diced tomatoes
- 5 1/8 ounces canned whole kernel corn
- 2 tsp. taco seasoning
- 3 tsp. ranch dressing mix
- 1/8 tsp. pepper
- 1/3 tsp. salt
- ½ C. diced onion
- 1 C. cooked ground beef

How it's made:

- Pour all recipe components into the instant pot.
- Cover and cook 10 minutes on MANUAL. Naturally release pressure for 5 minutes. Serve with favorite toppings.

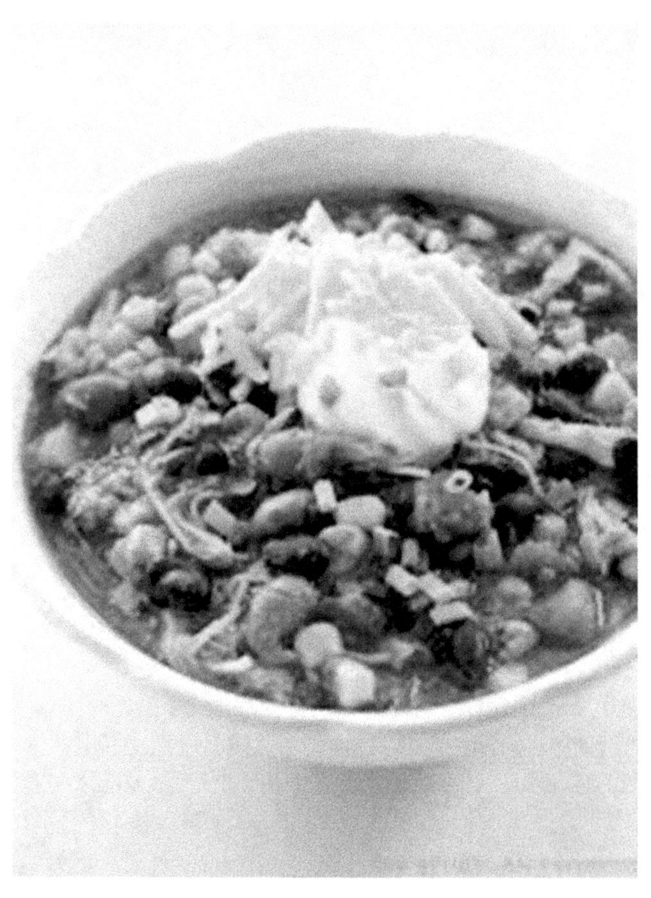

Lasagna Soup

What's in it:

- 1 C. ricotta cheese
- 1 C. shredded mozzarella cheese
- Pinch of oregano
- Pinch of salt
- 1 ½ C. uncooked noodles
- 1 jar spaghetti sauce
- 40 ounces chicken stock
- 1 C. diced tomatoes
- ½ diced onion
- 1 pound ground turkey

How it's made:

- Sauté onions and beef in instant pot.
- Add all recipe components minus cheeses.
- Cook 4 minutes on MANUAL. Perform natural release.
- Top with mozzarella and ricotta cheeses.

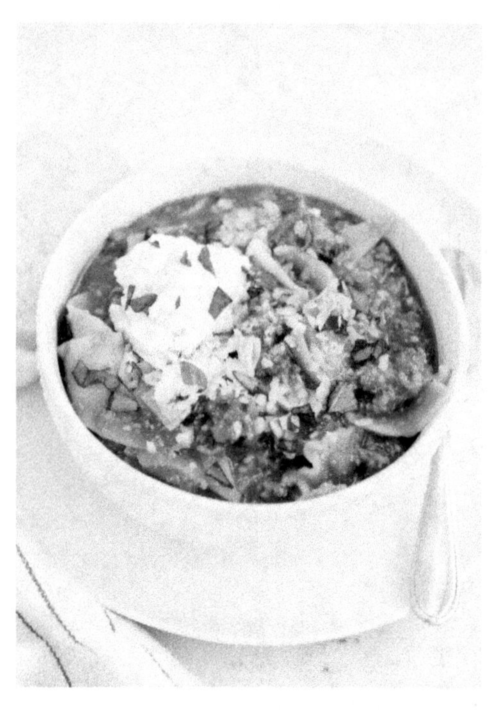

Stuffed Green Pepper Soup

What's in it:

- 2 C. cauliflower rice
- 2 diced green bell peppers
- 1 diced onion
- 3 C. low-sodium beef broth
- 2 C. tomato juice
- 1 28-ounce can diced tomatoes
- 1 clove of garlic
- 1 pound browned ground beef (preferably grass-fed)

How it's made:

- Brown beef and garlic together 2 minutes in instant pot.
  Pour in remaining ingredients into the instant pot. Combine well.
- Set to cook 20 minutes on HIGH PRESSURE.
- Add cauliflower rice to the instant pot and stir well. Enjoy!

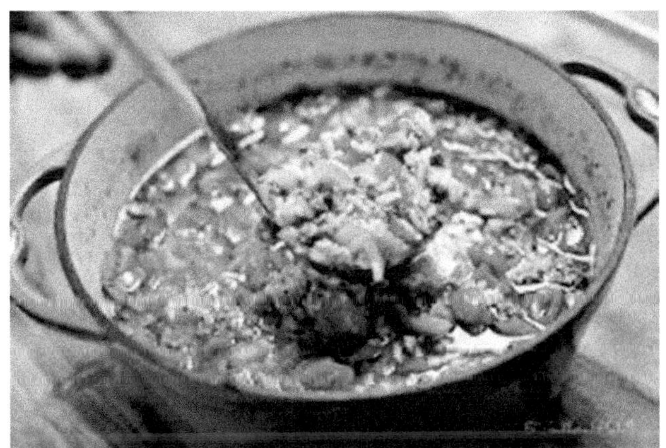

Egg Lemon Orzo Soup

What's in it:

- Juice of 2 lemons
- 3 eggs
- ¾ C. uncooked orzo
- 6 C. low-sodium chicken broth

How it's made:

- Pour orzo and chicken broth into the instant pot. Cook 5 minutes on MANUAL. Perform a quick release. Remove lid and hit SAUTE button.
- As broth and orzo cooks, stir lemon juice and eggs together.
- Gradually add broth into lemon-egg mixture. Stir 60 seconds.
- Pour mixture back into the instant pot. Stir constantly 3 minutes. When mixture begins to bubble, turn off the instant pot.
- Spoon mixture into bowls and garnish with feta cheese.

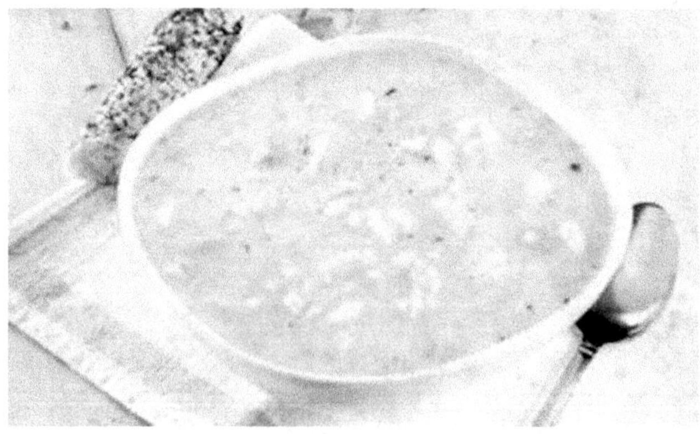

Split Pea Soup

What's in it:

- 1 C. diced ham
- 1 tsp. garlic powder
- 1 ½ tsp. salt
- 2 tbsp. olive oil
- 2 sliced celery stalks
- 2 sliced carrots
- ½ diced onion
- 2 C. dry split peas
- 40 ounces vegetable stock

How it's made:

- Sauté onions and ham in olive oil within instant pot till onions become soft.
- Pour in remaining recipe components into the instant pot.
- Close and cook 17 minutes on MANUAL. Perform quick release.
- Allow to sit for soup to become a bit thicken before serving. Top with cheese of choice if you desire.

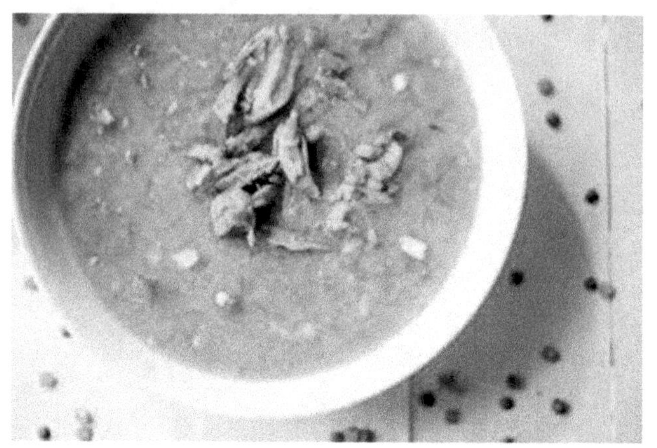

Butternut Squash and Apple Soup

What's in it:

- Olive oil
- 4 C. chicken broth
- Ginger powder
- 1 peeled/cut apple of choice
- 1 peeled/cut butternut squash

How it's made:

- Cut up squash into chunks. Peel and cut up the apple into chunks.
- Push SAUTE on your instant pot and warm up oil. Cook squash 5 minutes till slightly browned.
- Pour in remaining recipe components into the pot.
- Cover and cook 10 minutes on HIGH PRESSURE. Perform quick release.
- With an immersion blender, blend mixture until smooth and creamy.

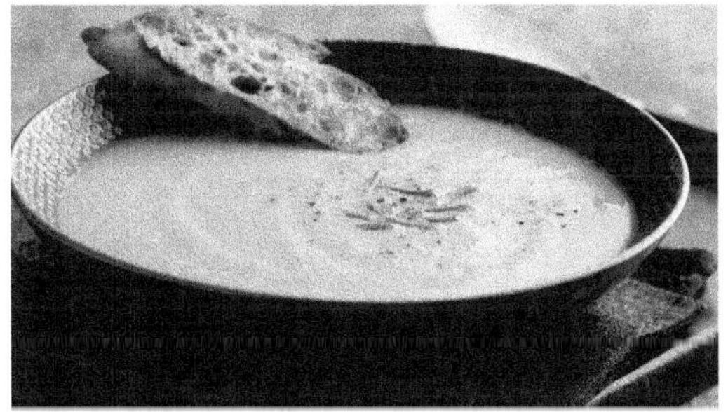

Chicken and Brown Rice Soup

What's in it:

- 1 tsp. coconut oil
- Pepper and salt
- ½ tsp. garlic powder
- 1 tsp. thyme
- 1 C. frozen peas
- 1 C. chopped onion
- 1 C. chopped celery
- 1 C. diced carrots
- 2 C. cooked brown rice
- 6 C. broth
- 2 frozen chicken breasts

How it's made:

- Sauté carrots, celery, and onions in coconut oil within the instant pot. Sauté till veggies become softened.
- Put chicken breasts into the pot over sautéed veggies.
- Add seasonings, peas, and broth. Mix in rice.
- Cover and set to cook 12-15 minutes on HIGH PRESSURE.
- Take out chicken and shred. Mix back into the instant pot and serve!

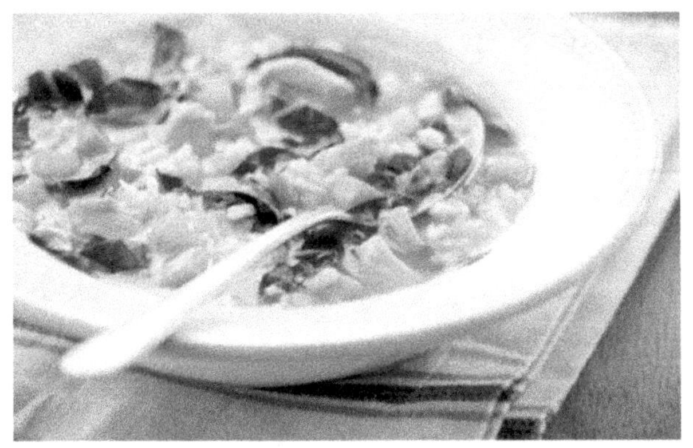

Side Recipes

Cilantro Lime Rice

What's in it:

- 3 ½ tbsp. lime juice
- ½ C. chopped cilantro
- 1 C. water
- Pinch of salt
- 1 C. uncooked white rice

How it's made:

- Pour rice into a strainer and rinse with water. Pour into the instant pot along with salt.
- Add water and stir well. Cover and press RICE.
- Allow pot to naturally release.
  Stir in lime juice, cilantro, and season with salt to achieve desired taste.
- Serve alongside a variety of dishes!

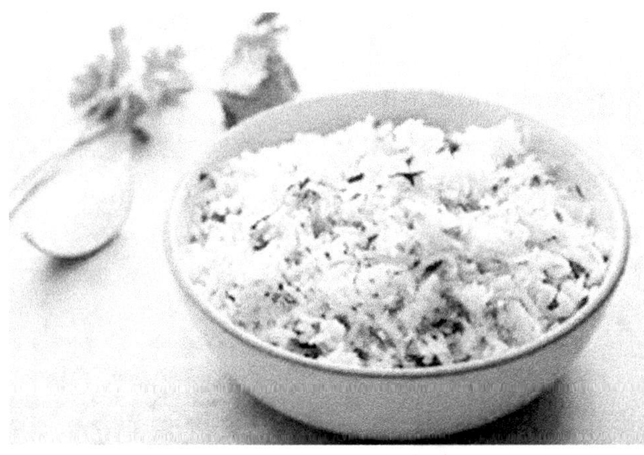

Cheesy Risotto with Spring Veggies

What's in it:

- 1 tsp. lemon peel
- 2/3 C. parmesan cheese
- 1 C. cherry tomatoes
- ½ tsp. salt
- 1 tsp. dried oregano
- 2 tbsp. lemon juice
- 3 C. low-sodium chicken broth
- 2 C. Arborio rice
- 2 tbsp. unsalted butter
- 3 cloves garlic
- 1 ½ C. asparagus
- ½ onion

How it's made:

- Sauté veggies with butter in instant pot. Sauté 3 minutes till softened. Press CANCEL to turn off sauté button.
- Add salt, oregano, lemon juice, and broth to the pot. Set to cook 6 minutes on HIGH PRESSURE.
- Perform a quick release when rice is done.
- Serve warm with lemon zest. Enjoy!

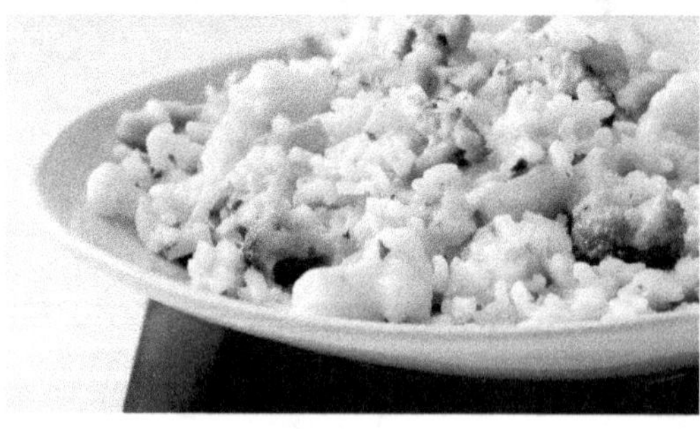

Pineapple Lime Rice

What's in it:

- 3 tbsp. lime juice
- ½ C. chopped green onions
- ¼ C. chopped cilantro
- ½ tsp. lime zest
- 4 tbsp. butter
- 1 C. water
- 8 ounce can crushed pineapple
- 1 ½ C. long-grain rice

How it's made:

- Place lime juice, lime zest, butter, water, pineapple, and rice into the instant pot. Set to cook 8 minutes on RICE setting.
- Perform natural release.
- Fluff rice and stir in green onions and cilantro. Enjoy!

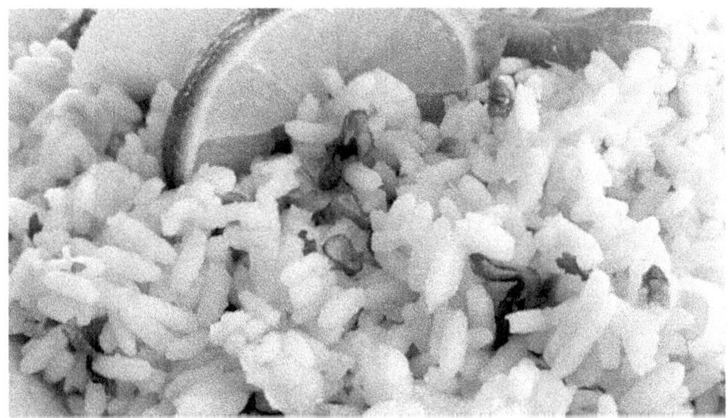

Instant Pot Scalloped Potatoes

What's in it:

- ½ tsp. dried thyme
- ½ tsp. garlic powder
- ¼ tsp. pepper
- 8 ounces shredded sharp white cheddar cheese
- ½ tsp. salt
- 3 tbsp. heavy cream
- 1 C. low-sodium vegetable broth
- 2 pounds small potatoes

How it's made:

- Peel and slice potatoes into ¼" thickness and pour into instant pot.
- Cook 1 minute on MANUAL. Perform quick release.
- Ensure your oven is preheated to broil.
- Pour potatoes into a baking dish.
- Pour all remaining recipe components into your instant pot, minus 2 ounces of cheese. Set to SAUTE and stir until creamy.
- Top potatoes with cheese sauce and sprinkle with reserved shredded cheese.
- Broil 4-6 minutes until browned and bubbly.

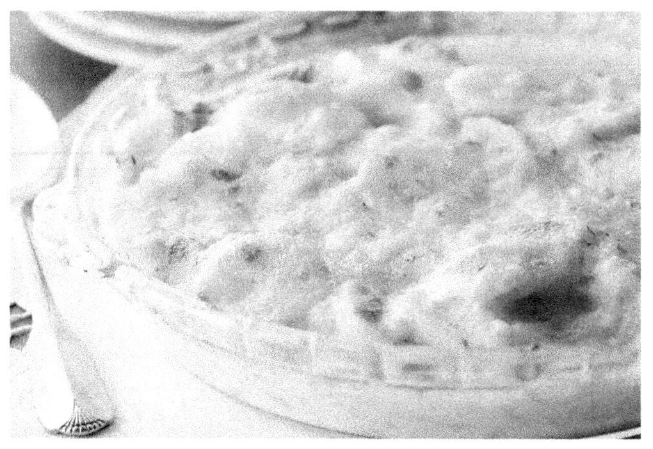

Spanish Brown Rice

What's in it:

- 1 tsp. salt
- 1 tbsp. cumin
- 2 ½ tbsp. chili powder
- ½ tsp. garlic powder
- ½ tsp. onion powder
- 2 tbsp. tomato paste
- 2 ½ C. water
- 2 C. uncooked brown rice

How it's made:

- Put water and rice into the instant pot.
- Set to cook 23 minutes on MANUAL. Perform quick release.
- Stir in remaining recipe components till combined. Enjoy!

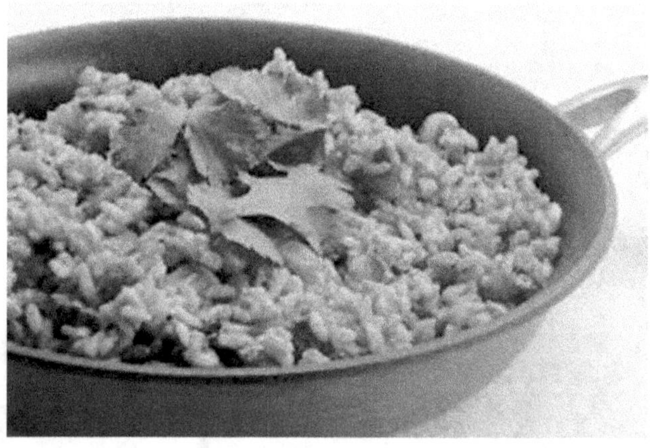

Stuffed Artichokes

What's in it:

- ¼ C. olive oil
- ¼ C. chopped parsley
- ½ tsp. pepper
- 1 tsp. salt
- 3 minced cloves garlic
- ½ C. grated parmesan cheese
- ¾ C. seasoned breadcrumbs
- 2 artichokes

How it's made:

- Cut steam and pointy tips from artichokes, as well as outer leaves.
- Place in a steamer rack within the instant pot. Pour in 1 ½ cups of water. Set to cook 4 minutes on STEAM. Perform quick release.
- Combine remaining recipe components together in a bowl as artichokes steam.
- With tongs, remove artichokes from the instant pot.
- Spread breadcrumb mixture in-between leaves of artichokes.
- Place back into the pot. Set to cook 8 minutes on HIGH PRESSURE. Perform quick release.
- Drizzle with olive oil and sprinkle with additional parmesan cheese when serving.

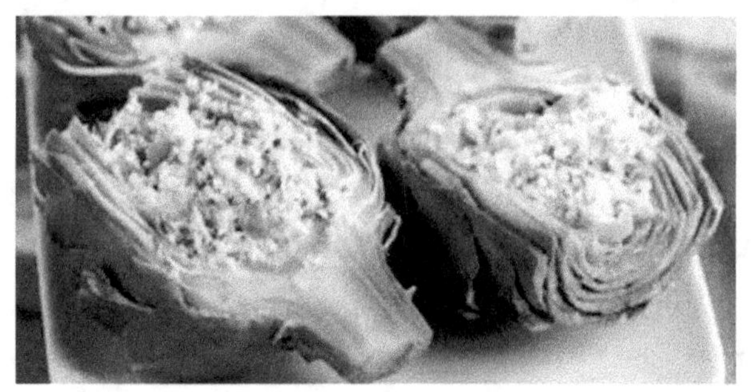

Instant Pot Mashed Potatoes

What's in it:

- ¼ C. sour cream
- Chopped chives
- Chopped dill
- Pepper and salt
- 1/3 C. half and half
- 2 tbsp. ghee
- 1 C. water
- 3 pounds russet potatoes

How it's made:

- Peel and cut potatoes into 1-inch chunks. Put into the instant pot.
- Pour just enough water to cover potatoes. Set to cook 7 minutes on MANUAL. Perform quick release.
- Drain potatoes and pour into a bowl. Add pepper, salt, and half and half. Stir well and then mix in sour cream, chives, and dill.
- Mash mixture with a potato masher till you reach desired consistency. Enjoy!

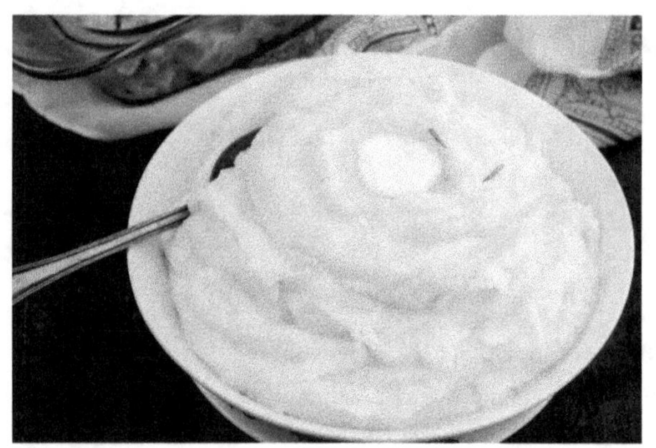

Instant Pot Cheesy Corn on the Cob

What's in it:

- 1 tsp. minced garlic
- 2 tbsp. grated parmesan cheese
- ¼ C. melted butter

How it's made:

- Put trivet into the instant pot and pour in 1 cup of water. Place corn cobs into the pot.
- Close and cook 2 minutes on MANUAL. Perform quick release.
- With tongs, remove corn cobs.
- Mix parmesan, garlic, and butter together and brush mixture liberally onto corn.

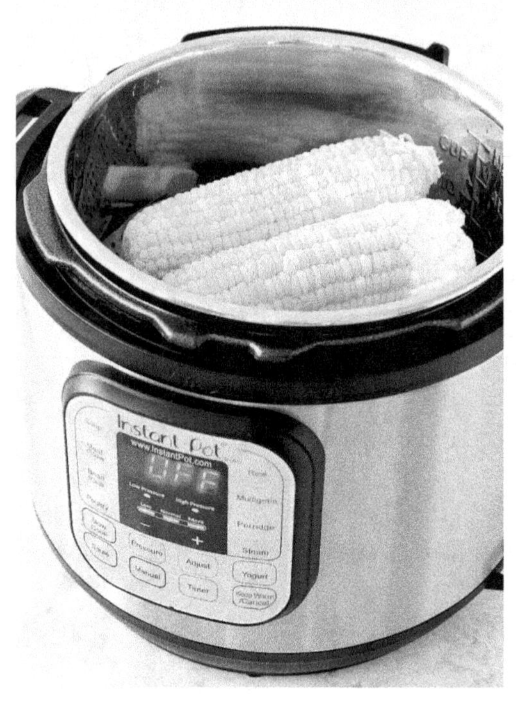

Cajun Spiced Zucchini

What's in it:

- 1 tsp. garlic powder
- 1 tsp. paprika
- 2 tbsp. Cajun seasoning
- ½ C. water
- 1 tbsp. butter
- 4 sliced zucchinis

How it's made:

- Place all recipe components into your instant pot. Gently stir to incorporate.
- Set to cook 1 minute on LOW PRESSURE. Serve!

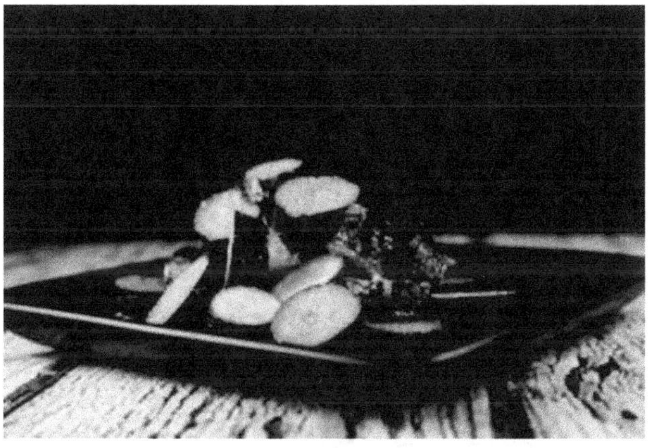

Instant Pot Refried Beans from Scratch

What's in it:

- 1 tsp. chili powder
- 1 tsp. cumin
- 1 tsp. salt
- 1 ½ C. pinto beans
- ½ onion

How it's made:

- Grease instant pot insert.
- Chop onion and add to pot.
  Rinse pinto beans and add them to pot with water and salt.
- Cook 35 minutes on HIGH PRESSURE. Perform natural release.
- Pour bean mixture into a blender. Add chili powder and cumin. Blend till you reach the consistency you desire.
- If you like chunkier beans, mash them instead of blending them. Enjoy!

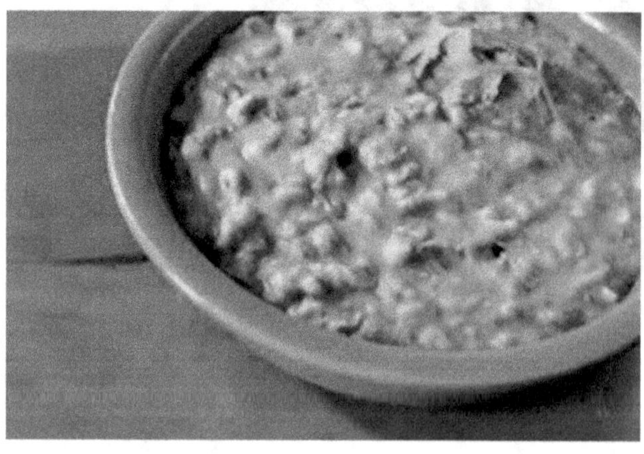

Instant Pot Lil' Smokies

What's in it:

- 4 ounces beer of choice
- 1 tbsp. honey
- 1 tbsp. white vinegar
- ¼ C. light brown sugar
- ½ bottle BBQ sauce
- 2 12-ounce cocktail sausages

How it's made:

- Put sausages into the instant pot. Then add beer, honey, vinegar, brown sugar, and BBQ sauce over sausages. Combine well to incorporate.
- Set to cook 1 minute on PRESSURE COOKER setting. Perform natural release for 5 minutes.
- If you want to thicken the sauce, set the pot to SAUTE for 5 minutes.
- Serve right away or set the pot to WARM to keep toasty till ready to devour.

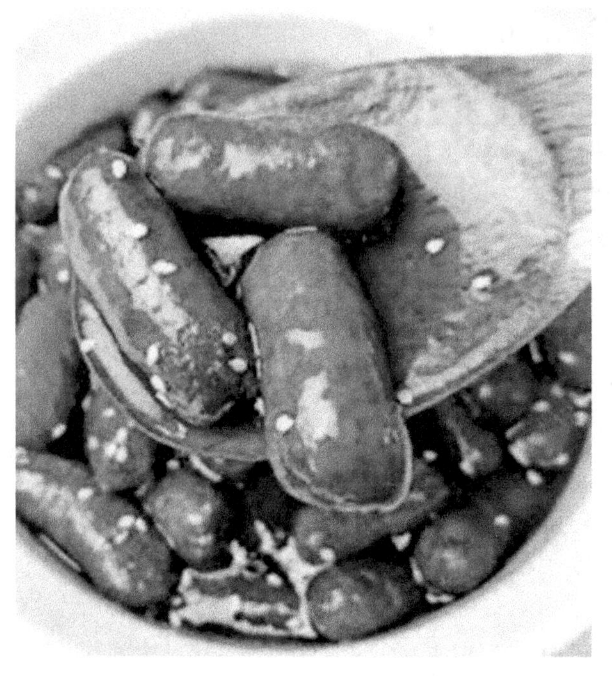

Pumpkin Risotto

What's in it:

- ½ C. canned pumpkin puree
- 1/8 C. white wine
- ¼ tsp. nutmeg
- ¼ tsp. pepper
- ½ tsp. salt
- 2 C. vegetable stock
- 1 C. Arborio rice
- ½ chopped onion
- 2 tsp. sage
- 2 tbsp. butter

How it's made:

- Melt butter in instant pot on SAUTE. Then add sage, fry for 1 minute. Remove sage mixture and set to the side.
- Add onions to pot and sauté 2 minutes. Then pour in rice and stir till rice is translucent and starts to toast.
- With white wine, deglaze the instant pot and then add vegetable stock, nutmeg, pepper, and salt. Combine well.
- Set pot to cook 9 minutes on HIGH PRESSURE. Perform quick release.
- Add in pumpkin along with a splash of vegetable stock.
- Top with parmesan cheese and serve garnished with fried sage.

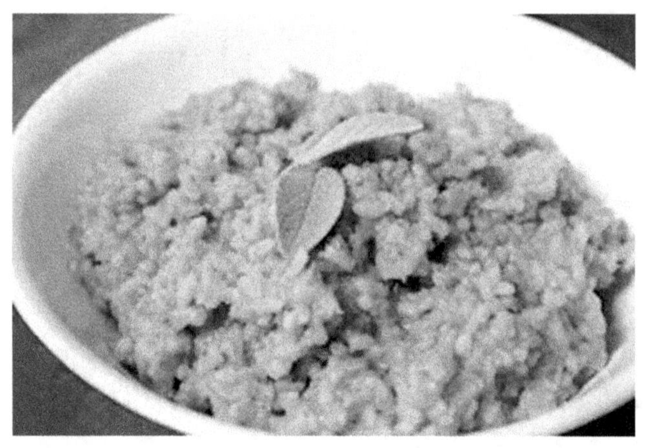

Snack Recipes

Instant Pot Yogurt

What's in it:

- 3 tbsp. plain Greek yogurt
- 1-gallon milk

How it's made:

- Pour all of the milk into your instant pot. Press YOGURT and adjust to BOIL. Cover and let milk boil 60 minutes.
- Stir milk and with a thermometer, make sure it reaches 180 degrees. If not quite there, use SAUTE and heat for a bit longer.
- Once the temperature reaches 180 degrees, take out the insert and set on the counter to cool to 110 degrees.
- Then add Greek yogurt, whisking into milk to combine.
- Press YOGURT and set to 8 hours.
- Chill in fridge and enjoy!

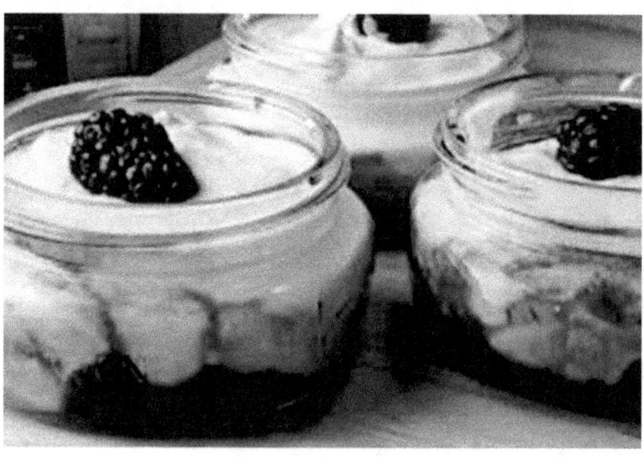

Apple Butter

What's in it:

- Pinch of ground cloves
- Pinch of grated nutmeg
- ½ tsp. cinnamon
- ¼ C. apple juice or water
- 5 ½ pounds cored/quartered apples

How it's made:

- Core and cut apples. Add to instant pot along with water.
- Set to cook 20 minutes on HIGH PRESSURE. Perform a natural release.
- With an immersion blender, puree mixture. Add spices and a bit of sugar if you desire.
- Cook uncovered 15-45 minutes by pressing SAUTE and adjusting to low.
- Stir occasionally until thickened.
- Store in a jar and chill.

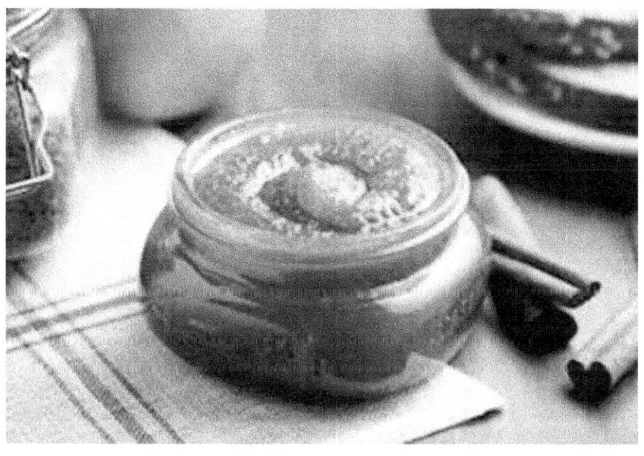

Garlic Hummus

What's in it:

- ½ - ¾ C. bean cooking liquid
- 1 ½ tsp. salt
- 3 tbsp. lemon juice
- 2 cloves garlic
- ½ C. tahini
- 6 C. water
- 1 ½ C. dried/rinsed chickpeas

Optional:

- Paprika
- Parsley
- Crushed red pepper

How it's made:

- Pour water and chickpeas into the instant pot. Cover and set to cook 40 minutes on MANUAL. Perform natural release for 15 minutes.
- Drain chickpeas and reserve cooking liquids.
- Process salt, garlic, lemon juice, tahini, and chickpeas in a food processor until creamy. Add ½ cup of reserved cooking liquid to achieve the consistency you desire.
- Season with pepper and salt and optional seasonings.

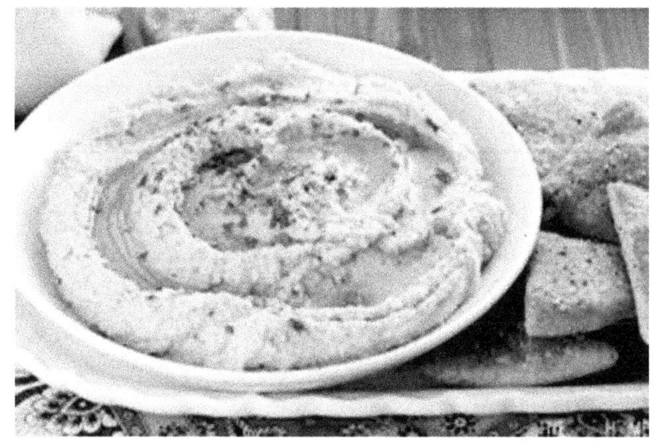

Instant Pot Salsa

What's in it:

- 4 tbsp. cilantro
- 3 tbsp. cayenne pepper
- 2 tbsp. garlic powder
- 1 tbsp. salt
- ½ C. vinegar
- 3 6-ounce cans tomato paste
- 1 C. jalapeno peppers
- 3 diced yellow onions
- 2 chopped green peppers
- 12 C. diced/peeled/seeded fresh tomatoes

How it's made:

- Mix together all ingredients in your instant pot.
- Cook 30 minutes on HIGH PRESSURE. Perform natural release.
- Let cool and store in an airtight container. Devour with chips, crackers, etc.

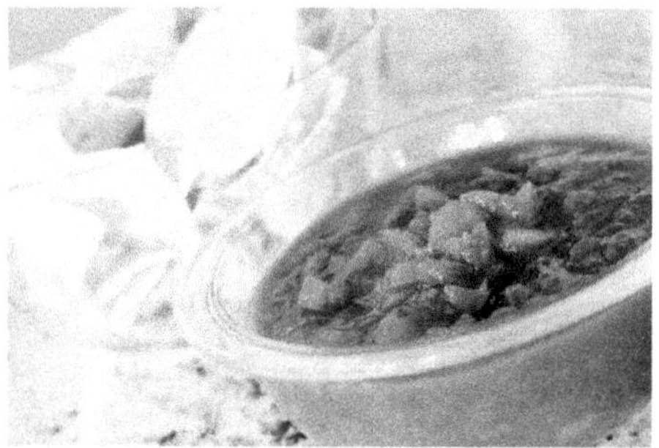

Buffalo Chicken Lettuce Wraps

What's in it:

- 1 sliced celery stalk
- ½ C. shredded carrots
- Large lettuce leaves
- ½ C. buffalo wing sauce
- 16-ounce low-sodium chicken broth
- 1 garlic clove
- 1 diced onion
- 1 celery stalk
- 1 boneless skinless chicken breast
- Ranch dressing, for serving

How it's made:

- Place buffalo wing sauce, garlic, celery stalk, onions, and chicken into your instant pot. Cover and cook on MANUAL 15 minutes. Perform natural release for 5 minutes.
- With a fork, shred chicken.
- Serve on top of lettuce leaves along with chopped celery, ranch dressings, and shredded carrots.

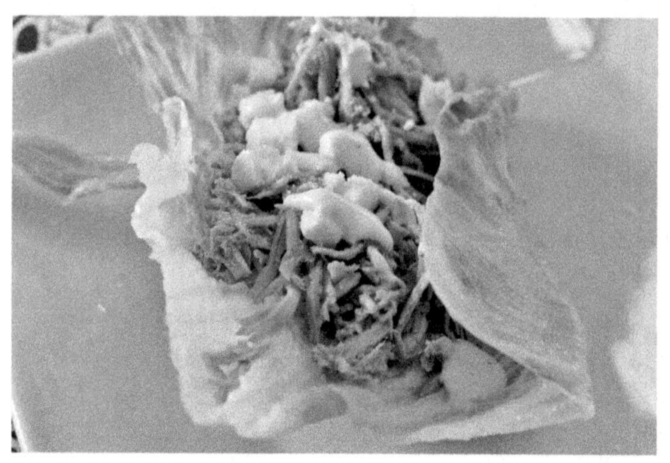

3-Minute Sugar-Free Pear Applesauce

What's in it:

- ½ C. water
- ¼ tsp. salt
- Juice of 1 lemon
- 1 tbsp. cinnamon
- 2 tbsp. ghee or coconut oil
- 6 pears
- 6 apples of choice

How it's made:

- Prep pears and apples by cutting them into chunks. Place into the instant pot.
- Add water, salt, lemon juice, cinnamon, and choice of fat to fruit.
- Cover and press MANUAL. HIGH PRESSURE should be lit up.
- Let your instant pot do its thing!
  Press WARM/CANCEL and walk away 15 minutes as it releases pressure.
- Spoon mixture into a blender and blender till smooth.
- Enjoy warm or cold!

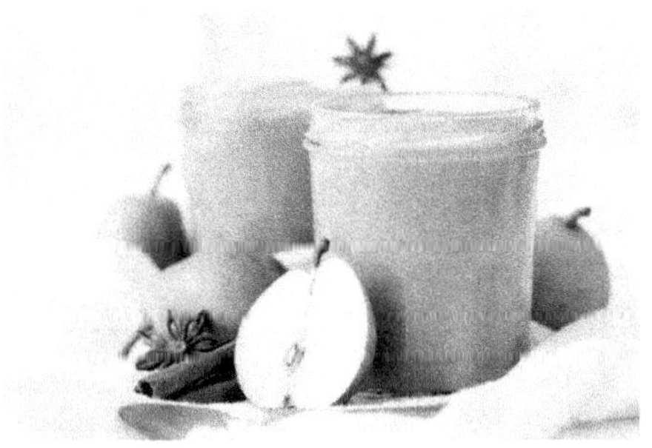

Candied Chickpea Cajun Trail Mix

What's in it:

- 6 ounces dried mango
- Pinch of salt
- Pinch of ginger
- ½ - 1 tbsp. spicy Cajun seasoning
- ½ C. pure maple syrup
- 2-3 tbsp. butter
- ¼ C. raw sunflower seeds
- 1/3 – ½ C. cashews
- 1 C. drained chickpeas
- 1 C. raw almonds
- 1 ½ C. raw pecan halves

How it's made:

- Pour in nuts, chickpeas, sunflower seeds, and ginger in the instant pot. Combine well.
- Sauté till thickened with butter. Add 1 tbsp. water if needed. Add in maple syrup and Cajun seasoning.
- Cook 10 minutes on MANUAL.
- Take out mixture and spread on a sheet. Bake 7-10 minutes at 375 degrees.
- Remove and let cool.
- Dice up mangos and stir into cooled trail mix and stir into mixture. Feel free to add more spices if you desire.

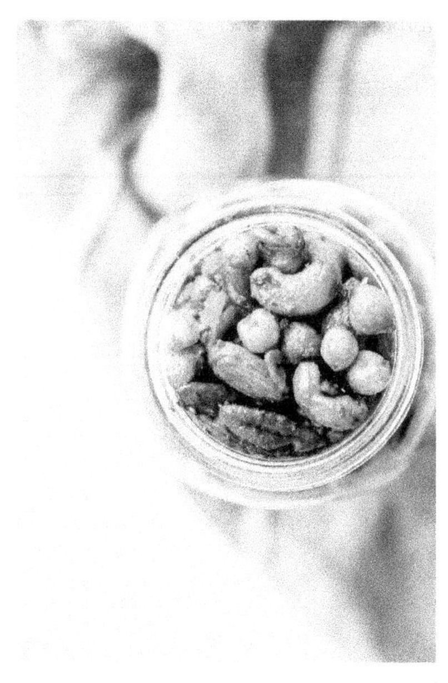

Perfect Instant Pot Eggs

What's in it:

- 1 C. water
- 4 eggs

How it's made:

- Put rack into the bottom of the instant pot. Pour in water and place eggs on rack.

- For *soft boiled eggs,* cook 3 minutes on HIGH PRESSURE. Perform quick release and run eggs under cold water till cool. Peel immediately.

- For *hard boiled eggs,* cook 5 minutes on MANUAL. Perform natural release for 5 minutes and then quick release. Run eggs under cold water and peel immediately.

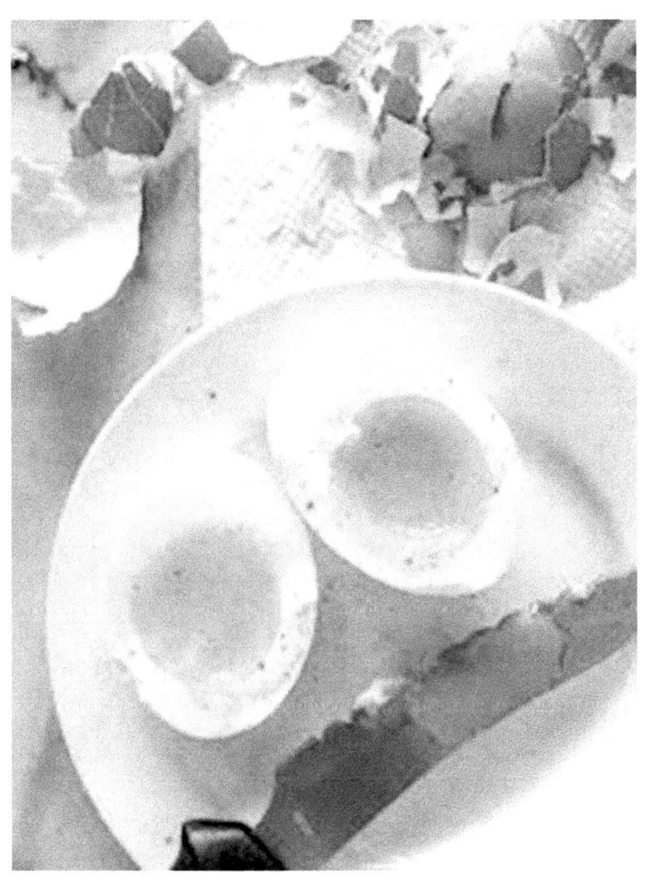

Instant Pot Rice Pudding

What's in it:

- Pinch of salt
- 1 can sweetened condensed milk
- ½ tsp. nutmeg
- 1 tsp. cinnamon
- 1 tsp. vanilla extract
- 1 C. long-grain rice
- 1 ¼ C. water
- 2 C. whole milk

How it's made:

- Rinse rice and drain.
- Add nutmeg, cinnamon, salt, water, and milk in your instant pot. Then add in rice and stir well.
- Close and cook 20 minutes on PORRIDGE setting. Perform natural release for 10 minutes/
- Push CANCEL and allow the pot to release remaining pressure. Stir in vanilla extract and milk until creamy.

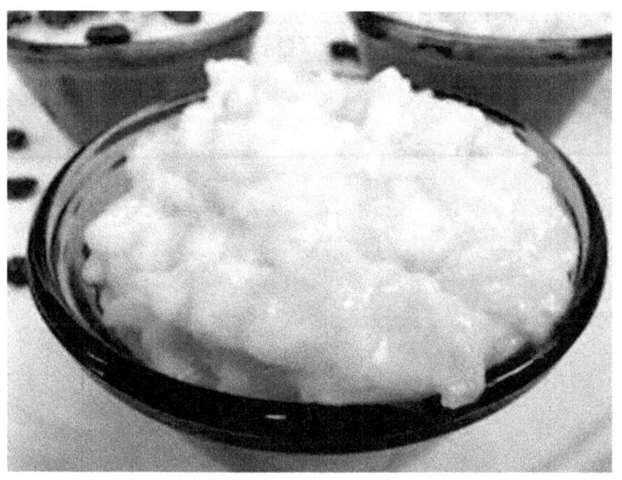

Instant Pot Low-Carb Hot Wings

What's in it:

- 1 tbsp. avocado oil
- Pepper and salt
- 3 minced cloves garlic
- 1 C. hot sauce
- 2 pounds chicken wings

Ranch Dip:

- 1 tsp. paprika
- ½ tsp. cayenne pepper
- 1 tsp. pepper
- 1 tsp. salt
- 1 tsp. dill
- 1 minced garlic cloves
- 3 chopped chives
- ½ C. chopped parsley
- 1 C. sour cream

How it's made:

- With pepper and salt, season wings. Pour hot sauce over wings.
  Marinate for at least 2 hours but preferably overnight.
- Pour wings, marinade and other recipe components into the instant pot.
- Set to cook 5 minutes on MANUAL. Perform quick release.
- To make ranch dip, mix all dip components together till creamy.

- Serve wings with dip and enjoy as a side or as a spicy snack!

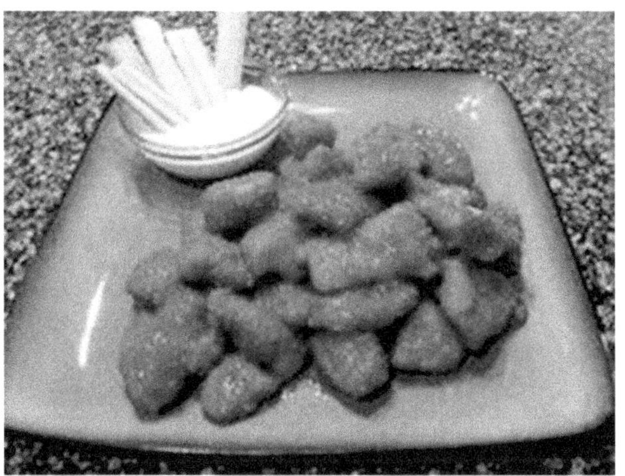

Dinner Recipes

<u>**Cracked Out Chicken**</u>

What's in it:

- 1 tsp. dill
- ½ tsp. parsley
- ½ tsp. pepper
- 1 tsp. onion powder
- ¼ C. Greek yogurt
- 1 tsp. garlic salt
- ¾ C. cottage cheese
- ¼ C. cheddar cheese
- 4 ounces turkey bacon
- 1 pound frozen chicken breast

How it's made:

- Put chicken into the instant pot along with 1 cup of water.
- Close and cook 12 minutes on HIGH PRESSURE. Perform natural release.
- As chicken cooks, cook turkey bacon and cut into cubes.
- In a blender, combine dill, parsley, onion powder, garlic salt, yogurt, and cottage cheese together until smooth.
- Drain and shred chicken within the instant pot. Pour dill dressing, cheddar cheese, and turkey bacon over chicken and combine well.
- Turn on the instant pot to SAUTE to melt cheese.

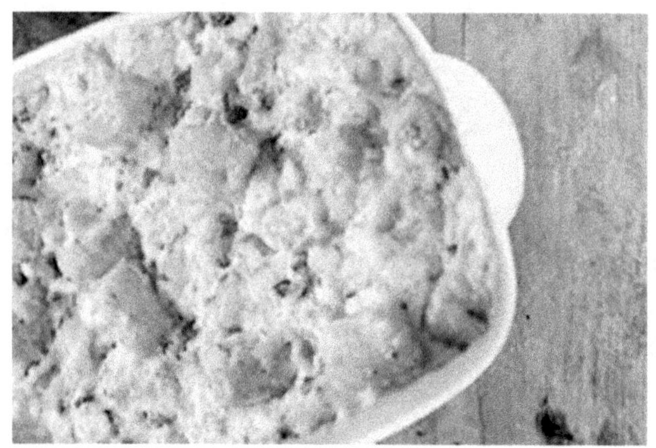

Sweet Potato Chili

What's in it:

- 1 tsp. cayenne pepper
- 2 chipotle peppers
- 1 tsp. cumin
- 1 tbsp. minced garlic
- 2 C. chicken stock
- 1 can drained black beans
- ½ C. crushed tomatoes
- 3 celery stalks
- 1 bell pepper
- ½ chopped onion
- 1-2 peeled/chopped sweet potatoes
- 1 pound ground turkey

How it's made:

- Set the instant pot to SAUTE and brown turkey. Drain grease.
- Add onions and garlic to turkey, cooking till soft.
- Then stir in cayenne pepper and cumin, along with chicken stock, sweet potatoes, crushed tomatoes, black beans, and chipotle peppers.
- Cover and cook 10 minutes on HIGH PRESSURE. Perform quick release.
- Turn instant pot to SAUTE. And add in celery and bell peppers. Simmer 5 minutes till celery becomes softened.
- Serve garnished with avocado, cilantro, and cheese. Enjoy!

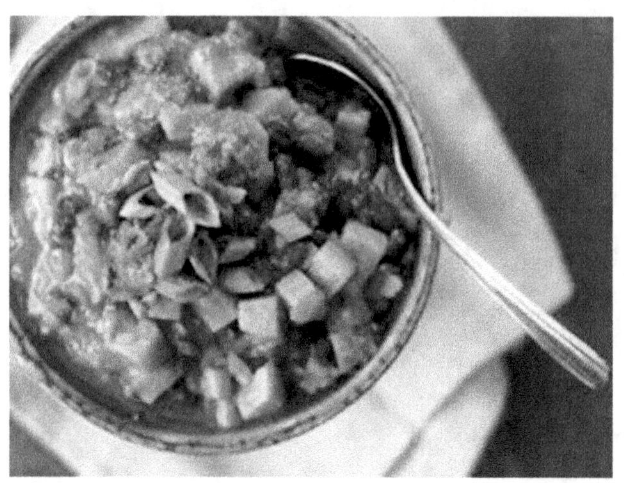

Shredded Mexican Chicken

What's in it:

- 1 tsp. liquid smoke
- ½ tsp. pepper
- 1 ½ tsp. salt
- ½ tsp. oregano
- ½ tsp. smoked paprika
- 1 tsp. garlic
- 1 tsp. cumin
- 1 tbsp. chili powder
- 14/5 ounce can diced tomatoes
- 4 tbsp. brown sugar
- 1-2 cans green chilies
- ½ C. mild salsa
- 1 tbsp. olive oil
- 2 pounds skinless, boneless chicken breasts

How it's made:

- Place chicken into instant pot and brush with olive oil. Pour all other recipe components over the top of chicken.
- Close and cook 27 minutes on MANUAL. Perform quick release.
- Shred chicken and place back into the instant pot.
- Cook 10-15 minutes to absorb the liquid.
  Serve with hot sauce!

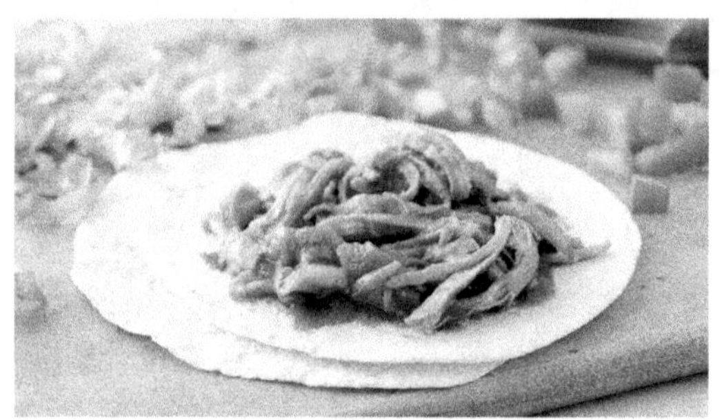

Swedish Meatballs

What's in it:

- 1 tsp. allspice
- 3 garlic cloves
- ½ tsp. pepper
- ½ tsp. salt
- 1 tsp. paprika
- 2 eggs
- ¼ C. chopped onion
- ½ C. crumbled whole grain crackers
- 1 pound ground turkey

Gravy:

- Pepper and salt
- ¼ C. parmesan cheese
- 1 tbsp. mustard
- 1 tbsp. amino
- ¼ C. parsley
- 1 ½ C. chicken broth
- ¾ C. Greek yogurt
- 2 tbsp. unsalted butter

How it's made:

- Mix all meatball components together. Form meatballs from the mixture.
  Push SAUTE on instant pot and melt butter. Place meatballs into pot and sear on all sides. Take out and set to the side.

- Pour in chicken broth and scrape the bottom to get browned bits up. Stir in mustard and amino. Then place meatballs gently back into the pot.
- Cook 5 minutes on HIGH PRESSURE. Perform natural release.
- Take out meatballs and allow the sauce to cool to room temp. Mix in yogurt until smooth and then parsley. Let sit so parsley softens.
- Pour sauce over meatballs and serve garnished with parmesan cheese.

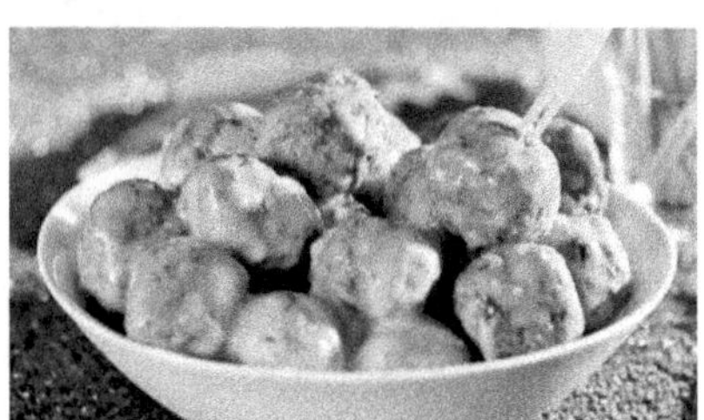

Tender Instant Pot Turkey Breast

What's in it:

- 3 tbsp. cold water
- 3 tbsp. cornstarch
- 1 sprig of thyme
- 1 celery stalk
- 1 onion
- 1 can turkey broth
- Pepper and salt
- 6 ½ pounds bone-in, skin-on turkey breast

How it's made:

- Liberally season turkey breast with pepper and salt. Make sure to get under the skin too.
- Place a trivet into the instant pot. Pour in thyme, chopped celery, chopped onion, and broth. Add turkey and cover. Cook 30 minutes on HIGH PRESSURE. Perform natural release for 10 minutes then quick release.
- Remove turkey and cover with foil.
- Strain fat from cooking liquid.
  Whisk cold water and cornstarch together. Pour in cooking liquid broth in with cornstarch mixture to the instant pot. SAUTE until thickened. Season with pepper and salt.
  Serve turkey with gravy.

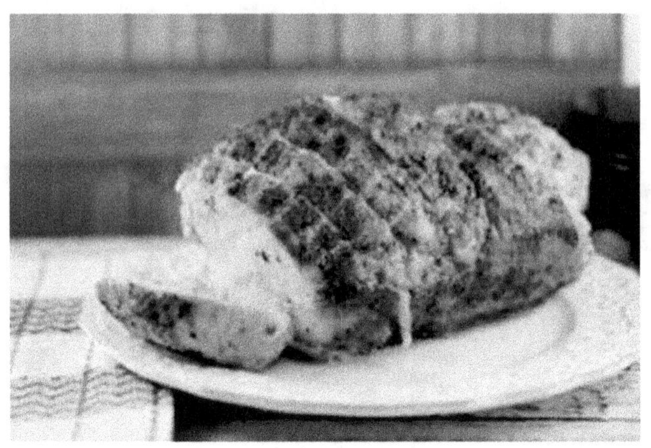

Instant Pot Spaghetti

What's in it:

- 1 can diced tomatoes
- 36 ounces water
- 1 jar spaghetti sauce
- 1 pound spaghetti noodles
- ½ tsp. garlic powder
- ½ tsp. onion powder
- ½ tsp. Italian seasoning
- 1 pound lean ground beef

How it's made:

- Set pot to SAUTE mode and place ground beef in. Cook with seasonings till cooked, breaking up as you go. Turn off the pot and drain grease.
- Break noodles in half and place on top of cooked meat mixture. Pour in water, diced tomatoes, and spaghetti sauce.
- Cook 8 minutes on HIGH PRESSURE. Perform quick release.
- Stir well before serving.

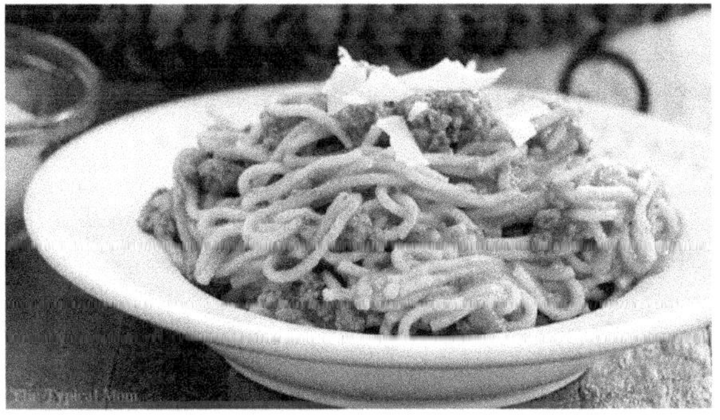

Avocado Lime Chicken Tacos

What's in it:

- Shredded cheese of choice
- Chopped lettuce, avocado, and tomato
- 1 tsp. garlic salt
- 1 tsp. cumin
- 1 sliced lime
- 3-4 chicken breasts

- Taco shells
- Favorite taco sauce

How it's made:

- Place chicken breasts with garlic salt and cumin into the instant pot. Set on HIGH PRESSURE to cook 8 minutes. Perform quick release.
- Remove chicken and shred with a fork.
- Spoon chicken mixture into taco shells and top with cheese, sauce of choice, avocado, tomato, and lettuce. Crunch away!

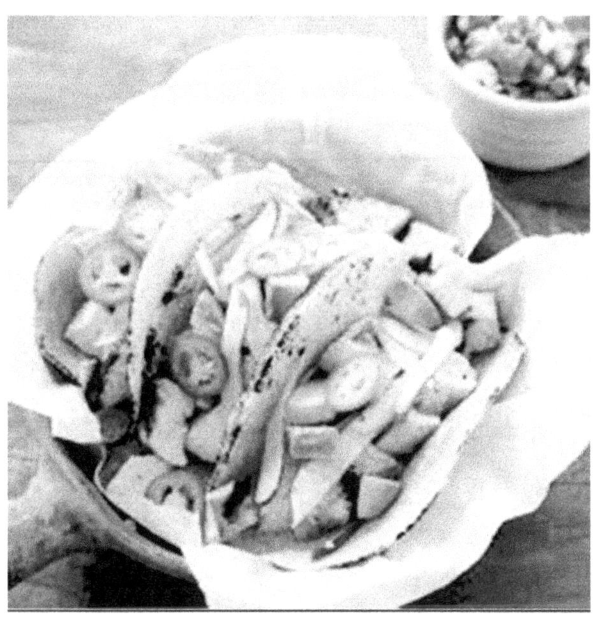

Low-Carb Pork Chops

What's in it:

- 1 tbsp. balsamic vinegar
- 1 C. mayo
- 1 tsp. nutmeg
- 1 tsp. garlic powder
- 3 boneless pork chops
- ½ C. oil
- 8 ounces brown mushrooms
- 1 yellow onion

How it's made:

- Wash and slice mushrooms. Peel and slice onion.
- Place pork chops into the instant pot along with onion and mushrooms.
- Whisk together vinegar, mayo, nutmeg, garlic powder, and oil. Pour over meat in instant pot.
- Cover and set to cook 20 minutes on HIGH PRESSURE. Perform natural release.
- Serve pork chops covered with onions, mushrooms, and some cooking liquid. Enjoy!

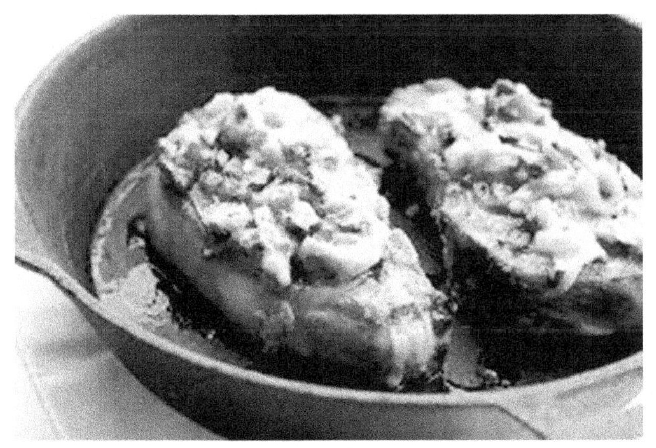

Low-Carb Pizza Casserole

What's in it:

- ½ tsp. onion powder
- ½ tsp. pepper
- 2 minced cloves of garlic
- ½ tsp. salt
- 1 tbsp. oregano
- ½ C. cheddar cheese
- ½ C. mozzarella cheese
- 1 package of pepperoni
- 1 pound ground turkey
- 2 C. crushed tomatoes

How it's made:

- Mix tomatoes and seasonings together. Pour ¼ of this mixture into bottom of the instant pot. Layer cheese, pepperoni, and turkey over the top. Continue this layering process till all ingredients are used. Cover and set to cook 6 minutes on HIGH PRESSURE. Perform natural release.
- Let cool 15 minutes, cut and serve!

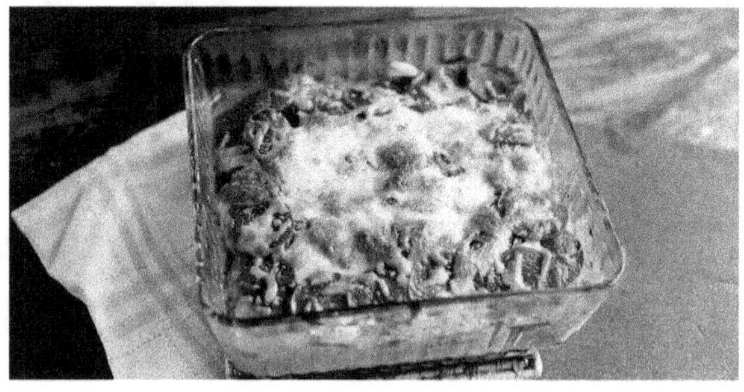

Coconut Shrimp

What's in it:

- ½ can unsweetened coconut milk
- 1 tsp. garam masala
- ½ tsp. cayenne pepper
- 1 tsp. salt
- ½ tsp. turmeric
- 1 tbsp. minced garlic
- 1 tbsp. minced ginger
- 1 pound shelled/deveined shrimp

How it's made:

- Pour 2 cups of water into the instant pot and top with a trivet.
- Combinc all rccipc components together within a vessel that fits into the pot. Cover it with foil. Place inside the instant pot.
- Set to cook 4 minutes on LOW PRESSURE. Perform quick release.
- Add more coconut milk if you desire. Enjoy!

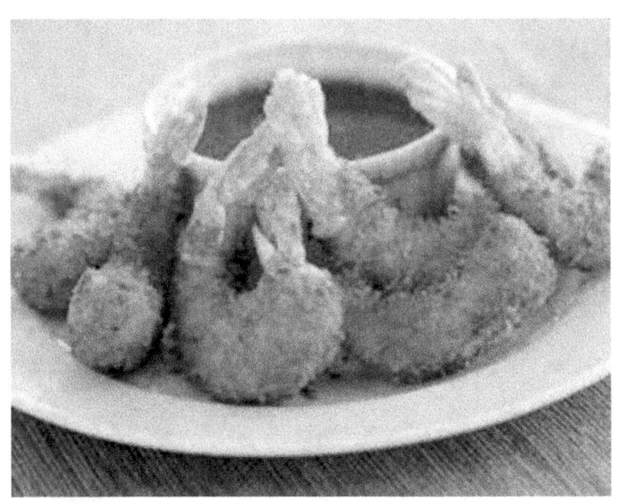

Dessert Recipes

Triple Chocolate Cheesecake

What's in it:

Crust:
- 4 tbsp. melted unsalted butter
- 20 Oreo cookies

Cheesecake:
- 1 tbsp. cocoa powder
- 1 tbsp. flour
- 1 tsp. vanilla extract
- 8 ounces 53-60% melted chocolate
- ¼ C. sour cream
- 2 egg yolks
- 1 whole egg
- ¼ C. sweetener of choice
- ¼ C. dark brown sugar
- 1 pound room temp cream cheese

Ganache:
- 3 ounces heavy whipping cream
- ¾ C. chocolate

How it's made:
- Grease spring pan. Pour 2 cups water into the instant pot. Create a sling out of foil, so lifting cheesecake in and out of the pot is easier.
- Combine butter with whole Oreo cookies in a food processor.
- Pour Oreo mixture into bottom of the pan and pat down gently. Freeze 10 minutes.
- In a clean food processor, combine cocoa powder, sweetener, dark brown sugar, and cream cheese together. Then add eggs and egg yolks. Mix well. Then

mix in sour cream and melted chocolate till well incorporated.
- Add flour and vanilla, mixing until creamy. Pour mixture over Oreo crust.
- Set pan into the instant pot. Set to cook 28 minutes on HIGH PRESSURE.
- Turn off and let sit 15 minutes. Perform quick release.
- Place cheesecake on a rack to cool. Chill overnight.
- To make ganache, warm whipping cream till it simmers and pour over chocolate. Then pour over cake and spread out evenly.
- Place in fridge to cool and serve!

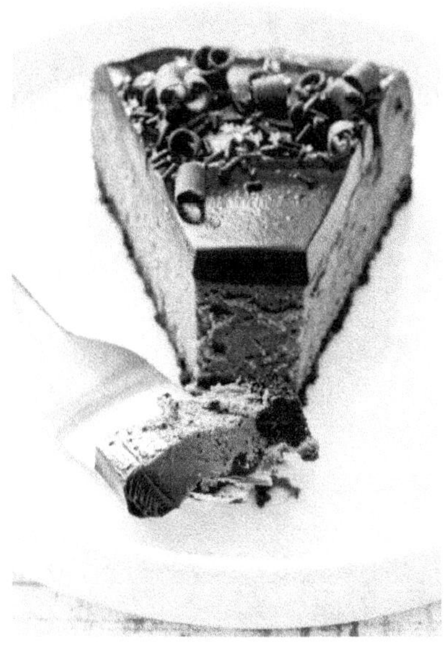

Raspberry Almond Coffee Cake

What's in it:

Crumble:

- 2 tbsp. chopped almonds
- 1 pinch of salt
- 1/3 C. low-carb brown sugar
- 1 ½ tbsp. sweetener of choice
- 2 tbsp. unsweetened shredded coconut meat
- 1/3 C. THM baking blend
- ¼ C. melted and cooled unsalted butter

Cake:

- 2 tbsp. apple cider vinegar
- ½ tsp. baking powder
- 3 tbsp. THM baking blend
- 3 tsp. THM super sweet blend
- 2 tsp. cream cheese
- 1 tsp. almond extract
- 2 whole eggs

- 1 C. frozen raspberries

How it's made:

- Mix together all cake recipe components together. Pour into a greased pan.
- Sprinkle berries over batter, keeping 6-7 aside for topping.
- Sprinkle crumble topping over batter and then top with reserved berries. With foil, cover pan.

- Place a trivet into your instant pot and pour in 1 cup of water. Place pan on top of the trivet.
- Cover and cook 30 minutes on HIGH. Perform natural release for 10 minutes.
- Let cool 10 minutes before attempting to cut and devour!

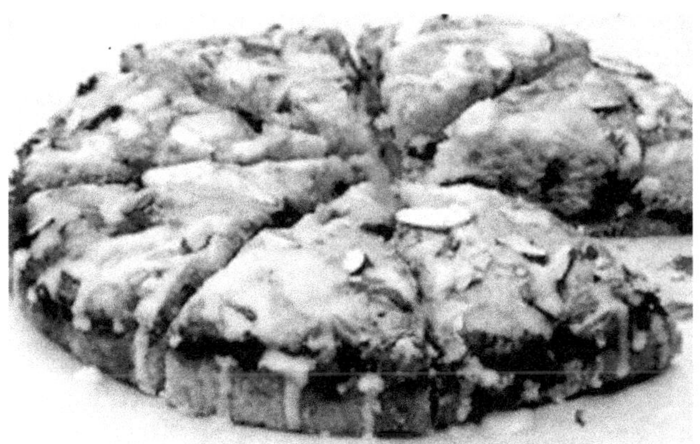

5-Minute Chocolate Pudding

What's in it:

- 1 tbsp + 2 tsp. grass-fed gelatin
- ¼ C. collagen
- 3-4 tbsp. cacao powder
- 1 tbsp. melted ghee
- 1 ½ tbsp. vanilla extract
- 1/3 C. honey
- 3 eggs
- 3 ¼ C. almond milk

How it's made:

- In a blender, combine almond milk cacao powder, vanilla, honey, and eggs together until smooth and well incorporated. Then add gelatin and collagen, blending 30 seconds till combined.
- Pour chocolate mixture into ½ pint jars, ensuring to leave ½" space between the lid.
- Pour 1 cup of water into the instant pot and place a trivet into the instant pot. Cover jars with lids and place upon trivet.
- Cover and press MANUAL. Set to 5 minutes.
- When the timer goes off, press WARM/CANCEL button. Turn to venting to manually release pressure. Carefully remove jars and allow to cool to room temp.
- Once cooled, shake them and chill them overnight.

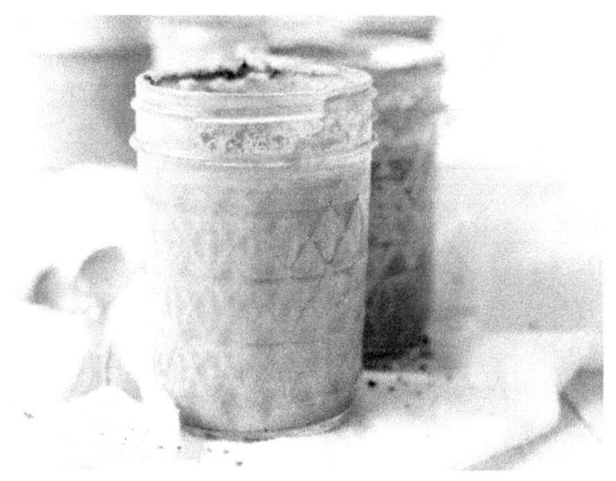

Chocolate Banana Cake

What's in it:

- 1 C. milk chocolate chips
- 1 tsp. vanilla extract
- ¾ C. brown sugar
- ¼ C. unsweetened applesauce
- ¼ C. melted butter
- 1 egg
- 3 ripe bananas
- 1 tsp. baking soda
- ½ tsp. salt
- ½ C. cocoa powder

How it's made:

- Mix salt, baking soda, cocoa, and flour together.
- Mash bananas and mix in egg, vanilla, brown sugar, applesauce, and butter.
- Fold dry mixture into wet mixture. Then fold in chocolate chips.
- Pour mixture into a greased dish that fits into the instant pot.
- Pour 1 ½ cups water into the instant pot and place trivet over water. Put cake dish upon trivet.
- Cover and set to cook 50 minutes on HIGH PRESSURE. Perform natural release for 8 minutes. Devour!!

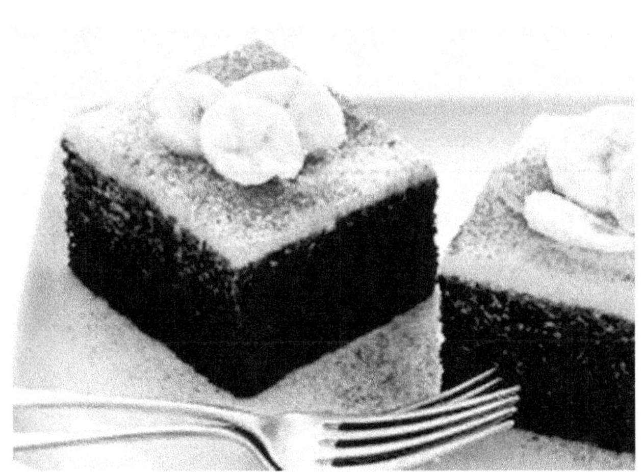

Peanut Butter Filled Brownies

What's in it:

- 1 tbsp. creamy peanut butter
- 1 ½ C. water
- 1 tbsp. diced walnuts
- 2 eggs
- ¾ tsp. baking powder
- ¼ tbsp. vanilla extract
- ¾ C. flour
- 1 C. sugar
- ¼ C. unsweetened cocoa powder
- 5 tbsp. melted butter

How it's made:

- Combine wet components in one bowl and wet components in another bowl. Then add wet and dry mixtures together, combining till incorporated.
- Grease a spring pan and line with parchment paper. Place peanut butter in the middle of the pan.
  Pour brownie batter on top of peanut butter and cover with foil.
- Put a trivet inside the instant pot and pour in 1 ½ cups water. Gently set pan into pot upon trivet.
- Set to cook 45 minutes on LOW PRESSURE. Perform a natural release.
- Let cool and put on a plate. Serve!

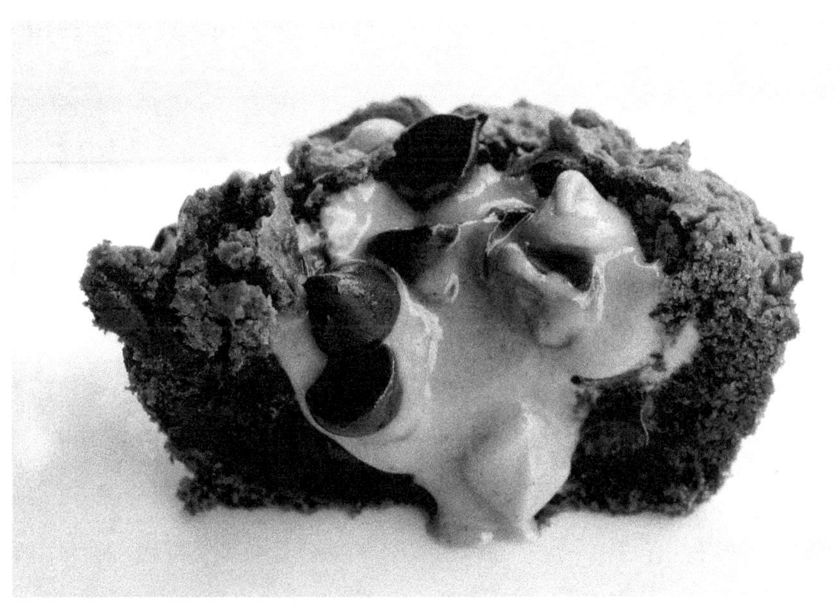

Instant Pot Carrot Cake

What's in it:

- 1/3 C. chopped toasted pecans
- 1/3 C. sweetened flaked coconut
- 1/3 C. grated carrots
- ¼ C. brown sugar
- ½ C. Splenda
- 4 tbsp. melted butter
- ¼ C. pineapple juice
- 3 tbsp. yogurt
- 2 eggs
- ¼ tsp. nutmeg
- ½ tsp. allspice
- ½ tsp. cinnamon
- ¼ tsp. salt
- ¾ tsp. baking powder
- ½ tsp. baking soda
- 1 C. all-purpose flour

How it's made:

- Mix all dry components together.
- Combine all wet components together. Fold wet and dry mixtures together. Fold in nuts.
- Grease spring pan.
- Pour 2 cups water into the instant pot. Place trivet over water and gently place pan upon trivet.
- Set to cook 32 minutes on MANUAL. Perform natural release for 10 minutes.
- Remove pan and let cool. Serve with vanilla ice cream!

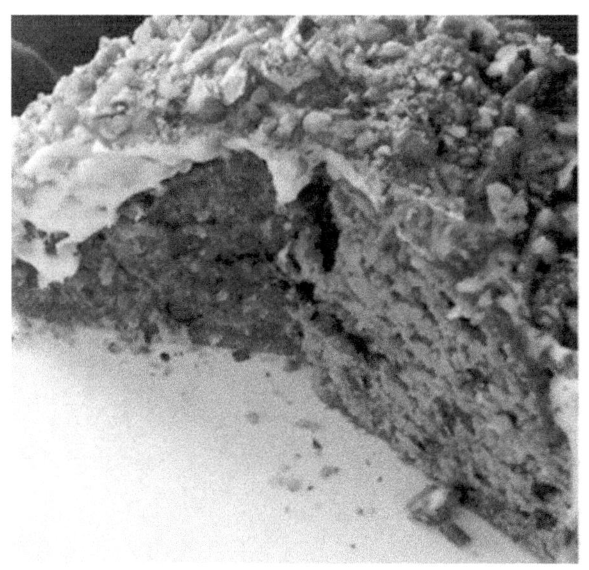

Chocolate Cobbler

What's in it:

- 2 ½ C. boiling water
- 2 tsp. vanilla extract
- ½ C. + 1 tbsp. cocoa powder
- 1 1/3 C. self-rising flour
- 1 C. Splenda
- ½ C. almond milk
- ½ C. melted butter

How it's made:

- Melt butter in instant pot on SAUTE.
- Turn off SAUTE and remove insert.
- Mix 1/3 cup Splenda, butter, vanilla, 2 tbsp. cocoa powder, milk, and flour together.
- Mix remaining Splenda and cocoa powder together and sprinkle over batter.
- Pour boiling water over, DON'T mix.
- Set pot to slow cooker mode and cook on HIGH 3 hours.
- Serve with ice cream!

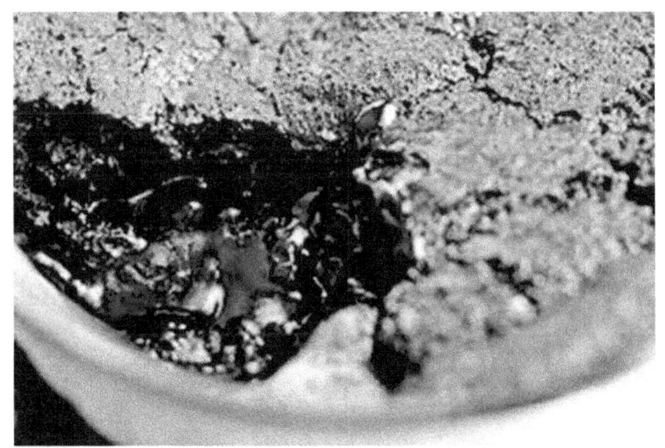

Baked Apples

What's in it:

- 2 tbsp. cinnamon
- ½ C. Splenda
- 1 C. apple juice
- 6 apples of choice

How it's made:

- Wash and core apples. Place apples into the instant pot and pour apple juice over them.
- Sprinkle apple mixture with cinnamon and Splenda.
- Cover and cook 8 minutes. Manually release pressure.
- Serve hot with a bit of cooking liquids over it with a dollop of whipped cream.

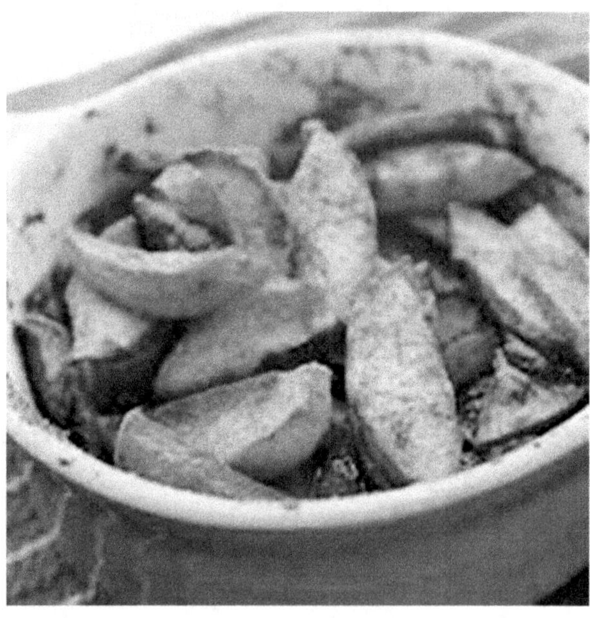

Lava Cakes

What's in it:

- 1 tbsp. cocoa powder
- ½ tsp. baking powder
- 1 tbsp. honey
- ¼ tsp. salt
- 1/3 C. rice flour
- 4 tbsp. coconut milk
- ¼ C. dark chocolate pieces
- 4 tbsp. ghee
- 2 eggs

How it's made:

- Melt dark chocolate and ghee together in the microwave for 30 seconds. Then mix in remaining recipe components into melted chocolate mixture.
- Grease 4 ramekins with coconut oil. Fill each ¾ full. When filling, place chocolate chunks in middle and top with remaining batter.
- With foil, cover chocolate filled ramekins.
- Pour 1 ½ cups of water into the instant pot and top with trivet. Place ramekins upon trivet.
- Cook 4-5 minutes on HIGH PRESSURE. 4 minutes will result in slightly gooey cakes while 5 minutes will result in more cake-like texture around the center.
- Use quick release method. Take out ramekins and turn upside down on serving plates.
- Serve hot with ice cream and/or whipped cream. Indulge!

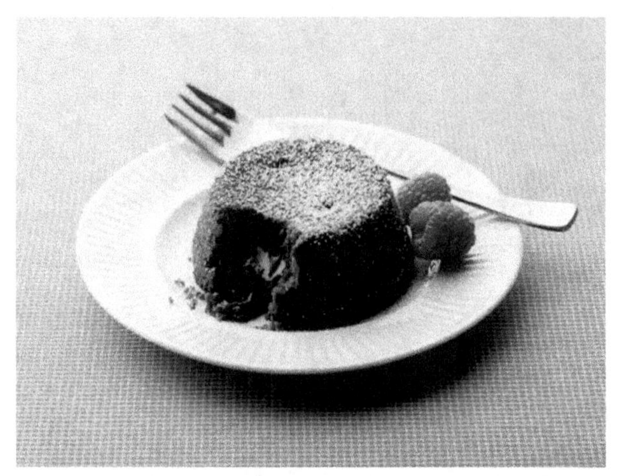

Instant Pot Peach Cobbler

What's in it:

- ½ tsp. cinnamon
- 5 tbsp. Splenda
- 1 tsp. vanilla extract
- 3 tbsp. melted butter
- ½ C. milk
- 2 1/3 C. baking mix
- ¾ C. water
- 3 tbsp. cornstarch
- 2 tsp. lemon juice
- ¼ tsp. cinnamon
- ¼ C. brown sugar
- ¼ C. Splenda
- Fresh peaches

How it's made:

- Slice peaches into wedges.
- Combine water, cornstarch, lemon juice, cinnamon, brown sugar, Splenda, and peaches together in instant pot.
- Combine vanilla extract, milk, baking mix together till thick. Spoon heaping spoonfuls of this mixture over peach mixture in pot.
- Combine remaining cinnamon and Splenda and sprinkle over peaches.
- Close and cook 15-17 minutes on HIGH PRESSURE. Naturally release pressure.
- Serve warm with a nice scoop of ice cream.

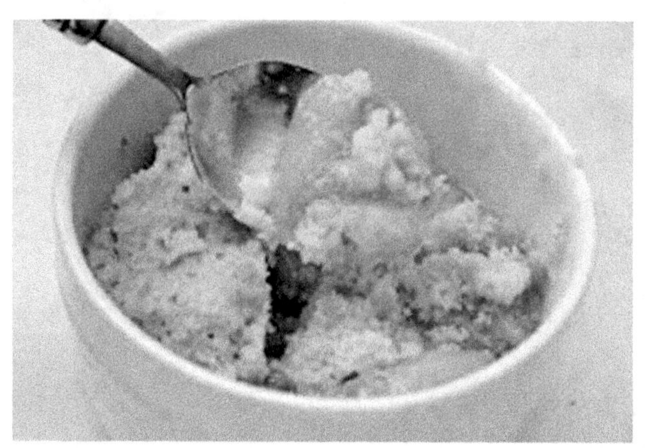

Drink Recipes

Skinny Pumpkin Spice Latte

What's in it:

- 1 tsp. vanilla extract
- 2 tbsp. stevia
- 2 tbsp. raw honey
- 1 tsp. chopped ginger
- ½ tsp. nutmeg
- 3 cinnamon sticks
- 1/3 C. pureed pumpkin
- 2 C. strong brewed coffee
- 4 C. unsweetened almond milk

How it's made:

- Mix together all latte recipe components into your instant pot.
- Cook 5 minutes on HIGH PRESSURE. Perform natural release for 10 minutes.
- Pour into mugs and serve topped with whipped cream. Add a sprinkle of nutmeg and a cinnamon stick for garnish, if desired.

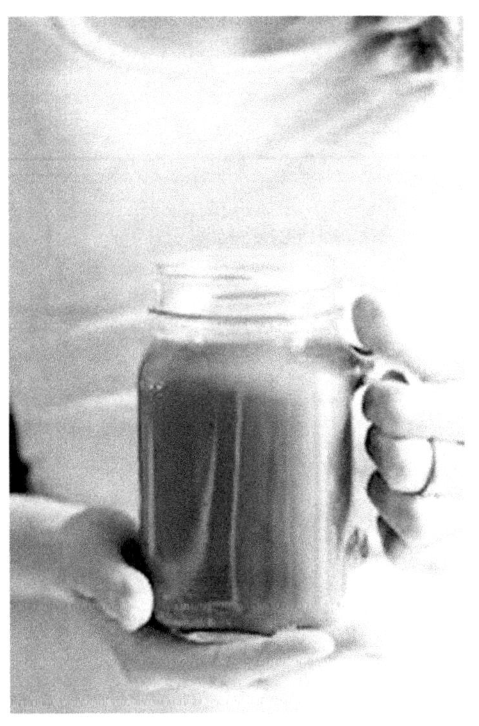

Hot Mulled Cider

What's in it:

- 1 thinly sliced apple of choice
- 2 thinly sliced oranges
- 2 whole cloves
- 2 whole star anises
- 2 cinnamon sticks
- 6 ounces lime juice
- 32 ounces cider
- 12 ounces Cointreau

How it's made:

- Place spices, fruit, lime juice and cider into the instant pot. Set to cook 3 minutes on HIGH PRESSURE. Perform quick release.
- Add Cointreau and cook 1 minute on HIGH PRESSURE. Quick release.
- Pour into mugs and garnish with an apple or orange slice and a cinnamon stick.

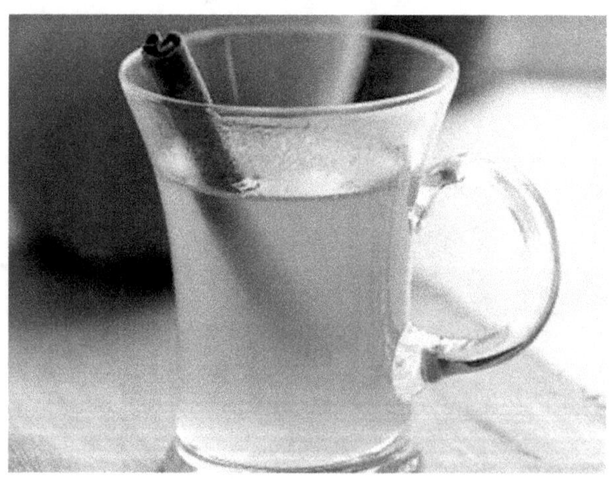

Instant Pot Ginger Ale

What's in it:

- 1-quart carbonated water
- 1 ½ C. granulated sweetener of choice
- 2 juiced lemons
- 1 pound fresh ginger (unpeeled and cut into cubes)

How it's made:

- In a food processor, blend lemon juice and ginger together until minced.
- Pour puree into the instant pot along with carbonated water and sweetener. Place lemon peel into the pot.
- Cook 30 minutes on HIGH. Perform naturally release.
- Allow to cool and strain. Then chill overnight.
- When serving, pour into glasses with ice with 2 tbsp. of ginger and a lime wedge. Enjoy!

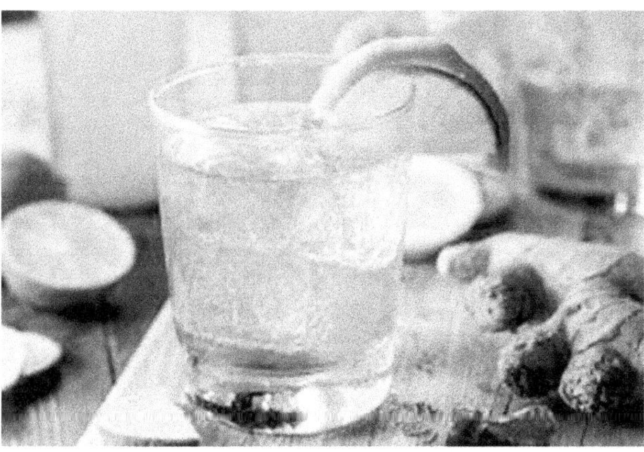

Horchata

What's in it:

- 1 cinnamon stick
- 6 tbsp. granulated sweetener of choice
- 32 ounces unsweetened rice milk

How it's made:

- Mix all recipe components together in the instant pot.
- Cook 4 minutes on HIGH PRESSURE. Perform natural release for 10 minutes.
- Chill and serve over ice and garnish with a sprinkle of cinnamon or a cinnamon stick.

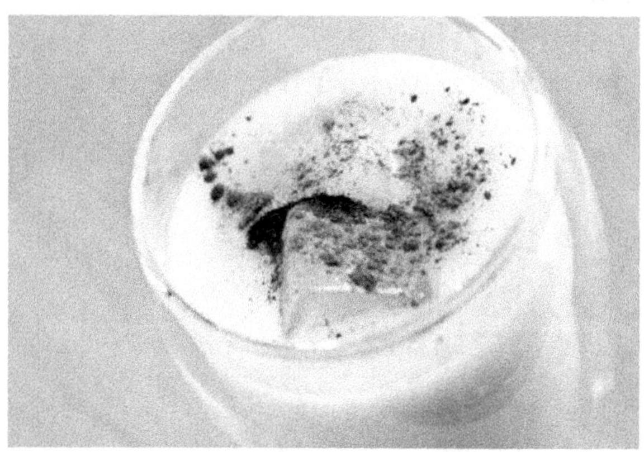

Limoncello

What's in it:

- 1 C. granulated sweetener of choice
- 1 ½ C. water
- 120-grain liquor of choice
- 2 half-pint canning jars
- 8 lemons

How it's made:

- Peel lemons and scrape off white portions. Split up peels among jars and fill jars with liquor, leaving ¾" of space on top. Cover with lids.
- Place a cup of water into the instant pot and place trivet over water. Gently put jars upon trivet.
- Cook 30 minutes on MANUAL. Perform natural release.
- Take out jars and allow to chill overnight.
- The next day, boil sweetener and water together to make a simple syrup. Let cool before mixing into liquor mixture.

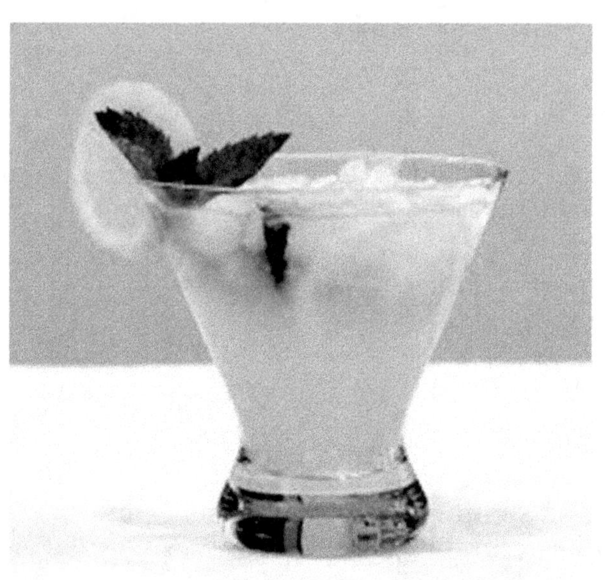

Spiced Apple Cider

What's in it:

- 7 whole cloves
- 2 cinnamon sticks
- 1" fresh ginger
- ¼ C. real maple syrup
- Zest and juice of 1 orange
- 2 ½ C. water
- 6 apples of choice

How it's made:

- Cut apples into quarters and remove the core.
- Add 2 ½ cups of water and apples in a blender. Blend until liquefied. Pour into a strainer to remove pulp.
- Pour apple juice into the instant pot. Mix in orange juice. Add more water if needed in order for the liquid to reach 5 cup mark.
- Add cloves, cinnamon sticks, ginger, maple syrup, and orange zest.
- Push SAUTE and allow mixture to heat to boiling.
- Then turn the instant pot off and cook on MANUAL for 10 minutes. Perform natural release for 15 minutes.
- Spoon cider through a strainer and drink right away!

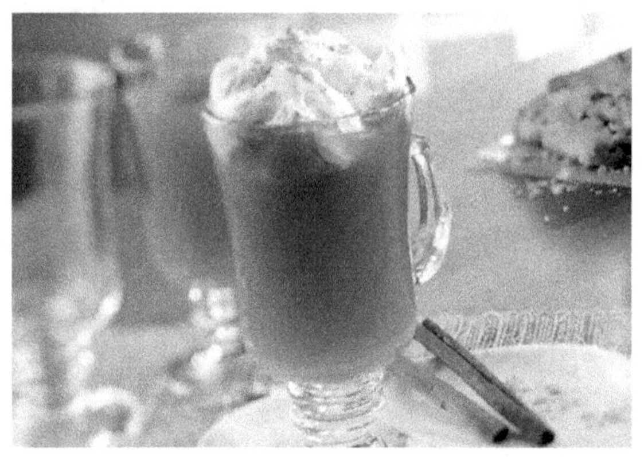

Zobo Hibiscus Tea

What's in it:

- Pineapple rind
- 1 tsp. grated ginger
- 1 C. granulated sweetener of choice
- 10 C. water
- 2 C. dried hibiscus petals (zobo leaves)

How it's made:

- Rinse hibiscus leaves with cold water.
- Add ginger, sweetener, and water into the instant pot. Stir till sweetener dissolves. Then stir in pineapple rind and hibiscus petals.
- Cover and set to cook 10 minutes on HIGH PRESSURE. Perform natural release for 30 minutes.
- Take out pineapple rinds. Pour into strainer and reserve strained liquid. Trash all solid ingredients.
- Pour into a container and chill.
- Serve over ice and sliced fruits of choice.

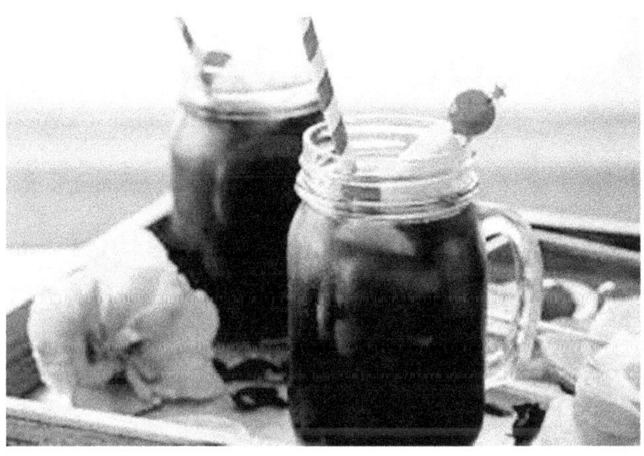

Instant Pot Iced Tea

What's in it:

- 1 C. granulated sweetener of choice
- 2 tsp. baking soda
- 10 tea bags
- 2 quarts water

Optional:

- Wild orange, peppermint, or lemon essential oils

How it's made:

- Place tea bags, baking soda, and water into the instant pot. Cover and cook 4 minutes on HIGH PRESSURE. Perform natural release.
- Uncover and stir on sweetener till dissolved.
- Pour mixture into a pitcher and chill. Mix in essential oils if using.
- Serve over ice with orange or lemon slices and fresh mint.

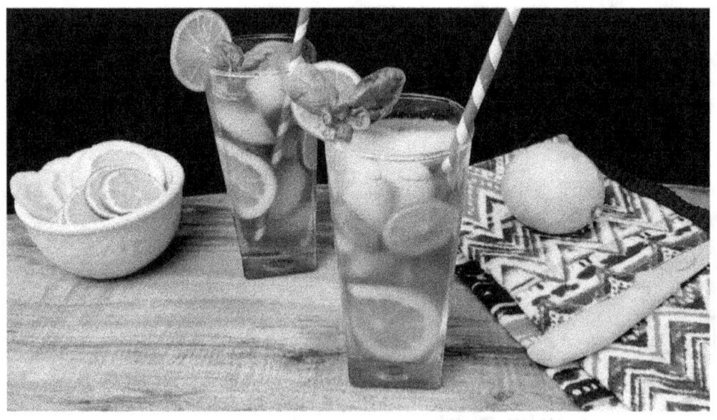

Conclusion

Thank you for reading through *Instant Pot Recipes.*

I hope that this book not only brought you comfort in knowing that you can utilize the convenience of the instant pot to your advantage when it comes to saving time and easing your health-conscious mind, but also that you can create a large variety of tasty meals in your very own kitchen!

I hope that you found this cookbook helpful in helping you to decide what to make to bring to your next family holiday or new ideas that are quick and easy to whip up on busy weeknights that the entire family will enjoy! Whether your goal is to save valuable time in the kitchen, to split your partnership with fast food places, or to simply learn more about cooking delicious meals all on your own, the instant pot is the perfect gadget for achieving all these goals and much more!

What are you waiting for? It is time to pick a few recipes to try out! Your taste buds are not going to be satisfied by this book collecting dust in your Kindle collection! It is time to start putting that instant pot to good use!

Did you find this book useful in any way? A moment of your time to leave an Amazon review would be much appreciated. Thank you and enjoy the array of recipes that you now have at your fingertips!